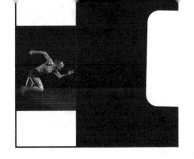

Student Workbook

to Accompany

Anatomy & Physiology
for Health Professions
An Interactive Journey

Fourth Edition

Bruce J. Colbert
Director of Allied Health
University of Pittsburgh at Johnstown

Jeff Ankney
Director of Clinical Education
University of Pittsburgh at Johnstown

Karen T. Lee
Associate Professor of Biology
University of Pittsburgh at Johnstown

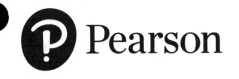

Senior Vice President, Portfolio Management: Adam Jaworski
Director, Portfolio Management: Marlene McHugh Pratt
Portfolio Manager: Derril Trakalo
Development Editor: Jill Rembetski, iD8-TripleSSS Media Development, LLC
Portfolio Management Assistant: Emily Edling
Vice President, Content Production and Digital Studio: Paul DeLuca
Managing Producer, Health Science: Melissa Bashe
Content Producer: Faye Gemmellaro
Editorial Project Manager: Ana Diaz-Caneja, Pearson CSC
Operations Specialist: Maura Zaldivar-Garcia
Creative Digital Lead: Mary Siener
Director, Digital Production: Amy Peltier
Digital Studio Producer, REVEL and e-text 2.0: Ellen Viganola
Digital Content Team Lead: Brian Prybella
Digital Content Project Lead: William Johnson
Vice President, Field Marketing: David Gesell
Executive Product Marketing Manager: Rachele Strober
Sr. Field Marketing Manager: Brittany Hammond
Full-Service Project Management and Composition: Pearson CSC, Blessy Zachariah
Inventory Manager: Vatche Demirdjian
Manager, Rights & Permissions: Gina Cheselka
Interior and Cover Design: Studio Montage
Cover Art: Dotshock/Shutterstock; Gehrke/Shutterstock
Printer/Binder: LSC Communications, Inc.
Cover Printer: LSC Communications, Inc.

Credits and acknowledgments for material borrowed from other sources and reproduced, with permission, in this textbook appear on the appropriate page within the text.

Copyright © 2020, 2016, 2011 by Pearson Education, Inc. All rights reserved. Copyright © 2014 by Pearson Education, Inc. or its affiliates. All Rights Reserved. Printed in the United States of America. This publication is protected by copyright, and permission should be obtained from the publisher prior to any prohibited reproduction, storage in a retrieval system, or transmission in any form or by any means, electronic, mechanical, photocopying, recording, or otherwise. For information regarding permissions, request forms and the appropriate contacts within the Pearson Education Global Rights & Permissions department, please visit www.pearsoned.com/permissions/.

Unless otherwise indicated herein, any third-party trademarks that may appear in this work are the property of their respective owners and any references to third-party trademarks, logos or other trade dress are for demonstrative or descriptive purposes only. Such references are not intended to imply any sponsorship, endorsement, authorization, or promotion of Pearson's products by the owners of such marks, or any relationship between the owner and Pearson Education, Inc. or its affiliates, authors, licensees or distributors.

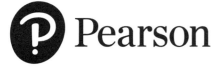

www.pearsonhighered.com

ISBN 10: 0-13-487917-1
ISBN 13: 978-0-13-487917-8

CONTENTS

Preface iv

Chapter 1 Introduction To Anatomy And Physiology: Learning The Language And Customs 1

Chapter 2 The Human Body: Reading The Map 11

Chapter 3 Biochemistry: The Basic Ingredients Of Life 21

Chapter 4 The Cells: The Raw Materials And Building Blocks 29

Chapter 5 Tissues And Systems: The Inside Story 39

Chapter 6 The Skeletal System: The Framework 51

Chapter 7 The Muscular System: Movement For The Journey 61

Chapter 8 The Integumentary System: The Protective Covering 73

Chapter 9 The Nervous System (Part I): The Information Super Highway 83

Chapter 10 The Nervous System (Part II): The Traffic Control Center 93

Chapter 11 The Senses: The Sights and Sounds 105

Chapter 12 The Endocrine System: The Body's Other Control Center 117

Chapter 13 The Cardiovascular System: Transport And Supply 127

Chapter 14 The Respiratory System: It's A Gas 139

Chapter 15 The Lymphatic and Immune Systems: Your Defense Systems 151

Chapter 16 The Gastrointestinal System: Fuel For The Trip 161

Chapter 17 The Urinary System: Filtration and Fluid Balance 171

Chapter 18 The Reproductive System: Replacement and Repair 181

Chapter 19 The Journey's End: Now What? 191

Answer Key 201

Copyright © 2020 by Pearson Education, Inc.

PREFACE

This workbook is designed to accompany the textbook *Anatomy and Physiology: An Interactive Journey for Health Professions*, Fourth Edition. Many of its features will allow you to work at your own pace and help you evaluate your progress throughout the course. Answers are provided in an answer key at the end of this workbook. There are features that will present a number of different ways to assess your progress as you journey through the text. Types of assessment features include:

Medical Terminology Review—This introductory section provides a review of key terms presented in the chapter.

Multiple Choice and Fill in the Blank—These review questions present an assessment to help test your knowledge of the chapter material.

Matching—This section asks you to match chapter terminology and concepts with appropriate definitions.

Short Answer—This feature helps you to think critically and apply the chapter knowledge.

Learning Activities:—Among the activities found in this section are engaging team projects, learning game ideas, and research topics.

Labeling—In some chapters, you are asked to identify anatomic structures and/or color a blank image with the appropriate structures. These illustrations correspond to those found in the textbook.

Crossword Puzzle—This feature will reinforce understanding of key terms and concepts.

Concept Maps—These maps provide an interactive visual overview showing the interrelatedness of the concepts within the chapter.

We hope this workbook helps make your journey through anatomy and physiology an enjoyable one.

INTRODUCTION TO ANATOMY AND PHYSIOLOGY: LEARNING THE LANGUAGE AND CUSTOMS

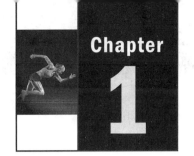

MEDICAL TERMINOLOGY REVIEW

Define the following terms.
1. Pathology: _____
2. Physiology: _____
3. Etiology: _____
4. Anatomy: _____
5. Diagnosis: _____
6. Prognosis: _____
7. Homeostasis: _____
8. Signs: _____
9. Symptoms: _____
10. Negative feedback: _____

MULTIPLE CHOICE

Circle the letter of the correct answer.

1. The study of structure is called:
   a. pathology.
   b. anatomy.
   c. physiology.
   d. cytology.

2. The study of tissue structure and function is referred to as:
   a. cytology.
   b. dermatology.
   c. histology.
   d. anatomy.

3. What is the study of function?
   a. Physiology
   b. Anatomy
   c. Pathology
   d. Cytology

4. The process of assessing the overall size and scarring pattern of the liver uses:
   a. macroscopic anatomy.
   b. microscopic physiology.
   c. macroscopic cytology.
   d. microscopic histology.

5. This system of measurement uses units that are multiples of 10:
   a. U.S. Customary.
   b. British Imperial.
   c. English.
   d. metric.

6. The science and study of the causes of diseases is called:
   a. anatomy.
   b. hepatology.
   c. diseasology.
   d. pathology.

7. What is a forecast of the probable course or outcome of a disease?
   a. Sign
   b. Prognosis
   c. Diagnosis
   d. Symptom

8. A disease-producing organism is called:
   a. harmless.
   b. pathogenic.
   c. pathological.
   d. inflammatory.

9. The period of time during which the signs or symptoms of a chronic disease disappear is known as:
   a. relapse.
   b. remission.
   c. prevention.
   d. exacerbation.

10. In the metric system, volume is expressed in:
    a. milliliters.
    b. kilograms.
    c. pints.
    d. cubic hectares.

11. The foundation of a word is its:
    a. prefix.
    b. root.
    c. suffix.
    d. etiology.

12. In the metric system, distance is expressed in:
    a. feet.
    b. kilograms.
    c. meters.
    d. liters.

13. During a hemorrhage, blood pressure falls and then the heart rate increases, which raises blood pressure. What is the name of this process?
    a. Positive feedback
    b. Metabolism
    c. Hemostasis
    d. Negative feedback

14. Any abnormality indicative of disease and objectively discoverable during examination of a patient is called:
    a. a syndrome.
    b. a symptom.
    c. a sign.
    d. septic.

15. Determining or identifying the nature of a disease, injury, or congenital defect is called a:
    a. sign.
    b. syndrome.
    c. prognosis.
    d. diagnosis.

16. Any subjective departure from the normal function or structure or sensation experienced by the patient or client is referred to as a(n):
    a. prognosis.
    b. diagnosis.
    c. symptom.
    d. etiology.

17. The study of disease is called:
    a. proctology.
    b. parasitology.
    c. pathology.
    d. psychology.

18. During breastfeeding, the harder and more frequently the infant suckles, the more milk is produced and secreted from the mammary glands and ducts. This phenomenon is called:
    a. metabolism.
    b. anabolism.
    c. negative feedback.
    d. positive feedback.

19. The medical term for outer layer of skin is:
    a. dermatitis.
    b. epidermis.
    c. hypodermis.
    d. paradermotomy.

20. A disease that spreads throughout a population or region would be considered:
    a. endemic.
    b. pandemic.
    c. hyperdemic.
    d. epidemic.

21. In the term *hypoglycemia*, its prefix is:
    a. hypo.
    b. glyc/o.
    c. emia.
    d. glycemia.

22. If *enter/o* means intestine, then what is the term for a painful, inflamed intestine?
    a. Enterology
    b. Paraenterotomy
    c. Enteritis
    d. Anenteromenorrhea

23. If *angio* means vessel, then what is the surgical repair of a vessel?
    a. Angioplasty
    b. Angiectomy
    c. Angiotomy
    d. Angiosurgery

24. Which of the following is considered a vital sign?
    a. Cyanosis
    b. Hypoglycemia
    c. Pulse
    d. Nausea

25. What occurs during anabolism?
    a. Building up
    b. Resting
    c. Breaking down
    d. Cooling

MATCHING EXERCISES

Match each term with the appropriate definition.

Set 1

_____ 1. phag/o
_____ 2. leuk/o
_____ 3. hepat/o
_____ 4. glyc/o
_____ 5. erythr/o
_____ 6. dermat/o
_____ 7. angi/o
_____ 8. gastr/o
_____ 9. oste/o
_____ 10. arthr/o

a. sugar
b. blood
c. vessel
d. joint
e. liver
f. red
g. bone
h. swallow
i. stomach
j. skin
k. intestine
l. white

Set 2

_____ 1. slow
_____ 2. pain
_____ 3. difficult
_____ 4. cutting into
_____ 5. within
_____ 6. surgical removal of
_____ 7. small
_____ 8. above normal
_____ 9. enlargement of
_____ 10. decrease or lack of

a. otomy
b. hyper
c. algia
d. peri
e. megaly
f. tachy
g. penia
h. an
i. brady
j. endo
k. ectomy
l. micro
m. dys

Set 3

___ 1. Patients with metabolic _____ may have hyperglycemia, hyperlipidemia, abdominal obesity, and high blood pressure.

___ 2. This is the name for the ability to control blood chemistry.

___ 3. A condition that presents with a rapid onset of signs and symptoms.

___ 4. Sweating when it is warm outside is an example of _____.

___ 5. Human body temperature = 98.6 is one example.

___ 6. Patient A feels tired and lethargic, her skin is flushed, and she has a rapid pulse. The attending health care professional believes the patient has water intoxication (hyponatremia), probably from the marathon run two days prior. In terms of the presented disorder/dysfunction, *the lack of electrolytes during the marathon* would be its _____.

___ 7. Patient A feels tired and lethargic, her skin is flushed, and she has a rapid pulse. The attending health care professional believes the patient has water intoxication (hyponatremia) probably from the marathon two days prior. In terms of the patient's condition, being *tired and lethargic* represents her _____.

___ 8. Patient A feels tired and lethargic, her skin is flushed, and she has a rapid pulse. The attending health care professional believes the patient has water intoxication (hyponatremia), probably from the marathon run two days prior. In terms of the presented disorder/dysfunction, *hyponatremia* is the _____.

___ 9. Patient A feels tired and lethargic, her skin is flushed, and she has a rapid pulse. The attending health care professional believes the patient has water intoxication (hyponatremia), probably from the marathon run two days prior. In terms of her condition, the rapid pulse would be its _____.

___ 10. This is the mechanism, also termed *vicious cycle*, by which the body continues the response or magnifies the response to a stimulus.

a. diagnosis
b. set point
c. negative feedback
d. acute
e. symptom
f. syndrome
g. etiology
h. homeostasis
i. sign
j. positive feedback

Set 4

_____ 1. a recording
_____ 2. one who specializes
_____ 3. condition of
_____ 4. form a surgical opening
_____ 5. extremities
_____ 6. through
_____ 7. upon
_____ 8. around
_____ 9. process of recording
_____ 10. one who studies

a. osis
b. logist
c. epi
d. acro
e. gram
f. ostomy
g. graphy
h. dia
i. ist
j. peri

FILL IN THE BLANK

Fill in the blanks to complete the following statements.

1. The medical abbreviation for *immediately* is:
   _____

2. The medical abbreviation for *nothing by mouth* is:
   _____

3. The adjustment made in the human body to maintain a stable internal environment by opposing the stimulus is:
   _____

4. The system of measurement most widely used in medical professions is:
   _____

5. Using the principles of medical terminology, what is *surgical removal of the kidney*? _____

6. Using the principles of medical terminology, what is the *study of the skin*? _____

7. Using the principles of medical terminology, what is *inflammation of the liver*? _____

8. Cholecyst/ means gallbladder. Using the principles of medical terminology, *the removal of the gallbladder* is termed:
   _____

9. The general term for the physiological process that maintains a stable internal environment is: _____

10. What is the cause of, or a reasonable explanation for, the manifestation of a disease? _____

11. The process of disease identification is called:
    _____

12. The prediction of a disease's outcome is called:
    _____

13. Cytology and histology are examples of
    _____ anatomy.

14. A(n) _____ is a specific group of signs and symptoms related to a particular disease.
15. Blood pressure, body temperature, and respiratory rate are examples of _____ signs.
16. Within the metric system, weight is often measured in _____.
17. A lab technician examining a slide for cancer cells would use a(n) _____ to see these tiny cells.
18. A young boy falls from his bike, breaking his arm. The pain and bruising are his _____.
19. A young boy falls from his bike, breaking his arm. The fall is the _____ of his injury.
20. A young boy falls from his bike, breaking his arm. A broken arm is his _____.
21. A young boy falls from his bike, breaking his arm. Surgery and a cast are the _____.
22. A young boy falls from his bike, breaking his arm. His _____ is that he'll be fine after several weeks in a cast.
23. Bill is very dizzy after a fall. Dizziness is a(n) _____.
24. If the word *hyperglycemia* means high blood sugar, what part of the word signifies blood? _____
25. A man is seriously injured in a car accident. He is bleeding severely, his blood pressure dropping. His heart races to try to bring up his blood pressure, but it continues to fall. His heart races faster and faster. What kind of feedback is affecting his heart rate?
_____

SHORT ANSWER

1. Contrast the terms *sign* and *symptom*.

_____
_____
_____
_____

2. Explain homeostasis.

_____
_____
_____
_____

3. How are anatomy and physiology related to each other?

   _____
   _____
   _____
   _____

4. Why is the metric system the measurement system of choice for science, medicine, and pharmaceuticals?

   _____
   _____
   _____
   _____
   _____

5. Explain how word roots, prefixes, and suffixes are put together to form complex medical terms.

   _____
   _____
   _____
   _____
   _____

LEARNING ACTIVITIES

1. Using a medical dictionary, see if you can determine what a word means by breaking it up into prefix, word root/combining form, and suffix. Each student should pick one word for the others to figure out.

2. Choose a disease and research its signs and symptoms on the internet. List them.

3. Pretend you are a surgeon. For as many surgeries as you can think of, try to determine the medical term for the surgery, using the roots, prefixes, and suffixes you already know. Use the internet or a medical dictionary to confirm your terms are correct.

4. Play "Medical Terminology Illustrator." One student draws a picture that represents a medical term while other students guess the correct term.

CROSSWORD PUZZLE

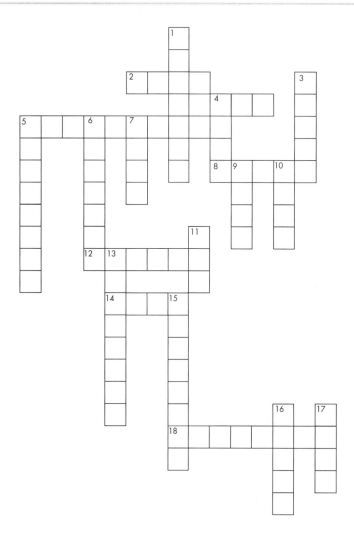

Across

2. metric system weight measurement
4. abbreviation for complete blood count
5. the study of function
8. word root meaning "bone"
12. suffix meaning "enlarged"
14. means "inflammation of"
18. feedback that resists a change

Down

1. the study of structure
3. prefix meaning "tissue"
4. word root for "cell"
5. feedback that enhances a change
6. subjective indicator of disease
7. means "condition of"
9. objective, measurable indicator of disease
10. within
11. prefix for "difficult"
13. cause of disease
15. ideal normal value
16. metric volume measurement
17. prefix meaning "around"

Name _____

CONCEPT MAP

Fill in the empty boxes with an appropriate term using the clues provided.

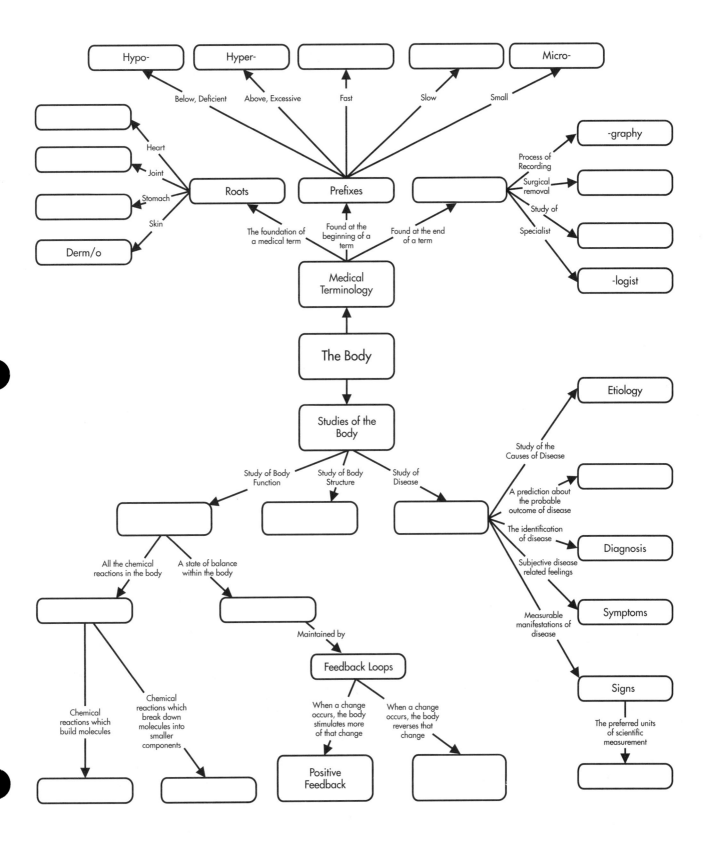

THE HUMAN BODY: READING THE MAP

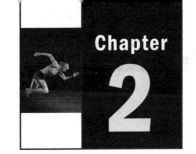

MEDICAL TERMINOLOGY REVIEW

Define the following terms.
1. Patellar: _____
2. Plantar: _____
3. Antecubital: _____
4. Femoral: _____
5. Axillary: _____
6. Carpal: _____
7. Cervical: _____
8. Lumbar: _____
9. Umbilical: _____
10. Thoracic: _____

MULTIPLE CHOICE

Circle the letter of the correct answer.

1. What structure separates the thoracic cavity from the abdominopelvic cavity?
   a. Navel
   b. Diaphragm
   c. Nipple
   d. Liver

2. A slice through the human body that parallels the long axis and extends from front to back, dividing the body into left and right halves, is called the:
   a. frontal plane.
   b. median plane.
   c. horizontal plane.
   d. mid-transverse plane.

3. Which is *not* part of the dorsal cavity?
   a. Oral cavity
   b. Vertebrae
   c. Cranium
   d. All of the above

4. The spleen is found in which abdominal quadrant?
   a. Right upper
   b. Right lower
   c. Left upper
   d. Left lower

5. Which term refers to the area anterior to the elbow, marked by a slight depression?
   a. Antecubital
   b. Anteradial
   c. Antebrachial
   d. Axillary

6. In anatomical position, how is the body positioned?
   a. Sitting with back straight, chest out, feet flat on the floor, and palms in neutral position
   b. Body erect, face and feet pointing forward
   c. Palms facing anteriorly, arms at the side
   d. b and c

7. Which plane divides the body and its parts into superior and inferior portions?
   a. Sagittal
   b. Midsagittal
   c. Cranial
   d. Transverse

8. Which is nearest to the point of origin?
   a. Distal
   b. Anterior
   c. Proximal
   d. Superior

9. The axillary region can be used to take temperature. Where is it?
   a. Armpit
   b. Ear
   c. Rectum
   d. Belly button

10. When referring to "toward the head," the correct term is:
    a. superior.
    b. dorsal.
    c. inferior.
    d. distal.

11. In reference to the antebrachium, where is the hand?
    a. Superior
    b. Distal
    c. Deep
    d. Proximal

12. A wound near the surface is:
    a. lateral.
    b. dorsal.
    c. ventral.
    d. superficial.

13. Where are the kidneys?
    a. Right and left upper quadrants
    b. Right and left lower quadrants
    c. Pelvic cavity
    d. Hypogastric region

14. In reference to the nose, where is the mouth?
    a. Superior
    b. Lateral
    c. Medial
    d. Inferior

15. A patient presents at the emergency department with a gunshot wound to her mediastinum. She is bleeding profusely. What major organ is probably damaged?
    a. Lung
    b. Heart
    c. Liver
    d. Stomach

16. Brown fat can accumulate in various parts of the body, including behind the knees. What is the clinical name of this area?
    a. Peroneal region
    b. Plantar region
    c. Patellar region
    d. Popliteal region

17. What is the back of the head called?
    a. Orbital region
    b. Buccal region
    c. Cervical region
    d. Occipital region

18. The dorsal cavity consists of which two cavities?
    a. Right and left pleural
    b. Right and left cerebral hemispheres
    c. Cranial and spinal
    d. Thoracic and pelvic

19. What is another term for *ventral*?
    a. Anterior
    b. Dorsal
    c. Posterior
    d. Cephalic

20. Carpal tunnel syndrome is due to inflammation of a nerve in this part of the body:
    a. wrist.
    b. neck.
    c. foot.
    d. lower back.

21. Many people who stand for long periods of time suffer pain due to plantar fasciitis. Where is their pain?
    a. Ankle
    b. Knee
    c. Sole of foot
    d. Hip

22. A patient recently diagnosed with breast cancer is scheduled for a lymph node biopsy to check for cancer spread into nearby lymph nodes. Which part of her body will be checked first?
    a. Abdominal
    b. Inguinal
    c. Lumbar
    d. Axillary

23. What structures are contained in the pleural cavities?
    a. Lungs
    b. Trachea
    c. Esophagus
    d. All of the above

24. The thoracic cavity contains the following organs:
    a. lungs, heart, and stomach.
    b. brain, spinal cord, and eyes.
    c. heart, lungs, and esophagus.
    d. stomach, spleen, and lungs.

25. The mediastinum is a subdivision of which cavity?
    a. Umbilical
    b. Epigastric
    c. Pleural
    d. Thoracic

MATCHING EXERCISES

Match each term with the appropriate definition.

Set 1

_____ 1. prone
_____ 2. superior
_____ 3. lateral
_____ 4. superficial
_____ 5. proximal
_____ 6. distal
_____ 7. deep
_____ 8. medial
_____ 9. inferior
_____ 10. supine

a. toward the surface
b. face up
c. caudal
d. to the front
e. away from the point of origin
f. away from the body's surface
g. away from midline
h. facedown
i. toward the point of origin
j. cephalic
k. to the back
l. toward midline

Set 2

_____ 1. buccal
_____ 2. mediastinum
_____ 3. abdominal
_____ 4. thoracic
_____ 5. dorsal
_____ 6. pelvic
_____ 7. umbilical
_____ 8. ventral
_____ 9. left hypochondriac
_____ 10. pleural

a. lungs, heart, and esophagus cavity (be specific)
b. spleen region
c. urinary bladder cavity (be specific)
d. pancreas quadrant
e. mouth cavity
f. lung cavity (be specific)
g. brain and spinal cord
h. liver cavity
i. lungs, liver, and uterus
j. between the lumbar regions
k. between inguinal regions
l. heart and esophagus cavity

Set 3

_____ 1. fingers
_____ 2. forearm
_____ 3. foot
_____ 4. breastbone
_____ 5. neck
_____ 6. wrist
_____ 7. thigh
_____ 8. lower back
_____ 9. eye area
_____ 10. mouth

a. femoral
b. pedal
c. sternal
d. antebrachium
e. orbital
f. digital
g. cervical
h. axillary
i. lumbar
j. carpal
k. oral

Set 4

_____ 1. antecubital
_____ 2. axillary
_____ 3. brachial
_____ 4. buccal
_____ 5. gluteal
_____ 6. nasal
_____ 7. patellar
_____ 8. plantar
_____ 9. pubic
_____ 10. thoracic

a. spray medications given here
b. checked for central cyanosis
c. warts here can be painful
d. collar for neck injuries placed here
e. can be used to take temperature
f. favorite place for body lice
g. where blood pressure is taken
h. an injection site
i. place where tendon reflex is checked
j. area used to draw blood
k. listen for heart sounds here

FILL IN THE BLANK

Fill in the blanks to complete the following statements.

1. The opposite of ventral is _____.
2. The common name for the buccal region is the _____.
3. The _____ test actually assesses for appendicitis by applying resistant force to a raised right leg.
4. In the thorax, the only cavities that are paired are called the _____ cavities.
5. The plane that divides the body into anterior and posterior sections is called the _____ plane.
6. The plane that divides the body into superior and inferior sections is called the _____ plane.
7. The female reproductive organs are located in a specific cavity called the _____ cavity.
8. Above the right inguinal region and below the right hypochondriac region is the _____ region.
9. Below the umbilical region is an area known as the _____ region.
10. The inguinal region is also called the _____ region.
11. When a person is lying on his back with the knees flexed and feet flat on the exam table, that is said to be the _____ position.
12. Medial to both the right and left hypochondriac regions is the _____ region.
13. In reference to the antebrachium, the brachium is _____.
14. In reference to the pleural cavities, the mediastinum is _____.
15. If the uterus is the point of origin and the vagina extends away from it, in clinical terms, the vagina is _____ to the uterus.
16. In medicine, "left" and "right" refer to the _____ (whose?) "left" and "right."
17. A patient has an injury to his lumbar vertebrae. Where is the injury? _____.
18. _____ is an imaging technique that uses sound waves to take real-time mages of the body.
19. To see a broken bone, the doctor would take a(n) _____.
20. To view the exact location of a tumor in 3-D, a(n) _____ is the best technique.

21. _____ is the highest density on an x-ray.
22. If a patient hits the back of his head, he may have injured his _____ region.
23. A cracked kneecap is a fractured _____.
24. A young girl falls head first down the basement steps. She has a severe laceration of her buccal region. The PA at the ED put the stitches in her _____ .
25. After a car accident, Gina complains of upper right quadrant abdominal pain. An MRI reveals internal bleeding caused by a lacerated _____. She is taken immediately to surgery.

SHORT ANSWER

1. Describe the clinical divisions or quadrants of the abdominal region.
   _____
   _____
   _____
   _____

2. List and explain planes of section.
   _____
   _____
   _____
   _____

3. Explain the anatomical position.
   _____
   _____
   _____
   _____

4. Explain in clinical and directional terms structures of the lower extremity from the hips to the toes.
   _____
   _____
   _____
   _____

5. List and explain the body cavities.

   _____
   _____
   _____
   _____

LEARNING ACTIVITIES

1. Buy several different types of fruits and vegetables at the grocery store. Cut each into sagittal, transverse, and frontal sections. How does each section differ?

2. Hide some "treasure." Write a treasure map using directional terms to guide other students to the treasure.

3. Select a body part. Using the internet, research the medical importance of that body part.

4. Play "Pin the Term on the Human." Make a cardboard cutout of a human shape. Pin the correct name on each part of the body. To make it harder, blindfold the player and use directional terms to guide him or her.

LABELING ACTIVITY

Shade each cavity with a contrasting color and list a major structure or organ contained in this cavity beneath the corresponding label. Use Figure 2–8 from your textbook as a guide.

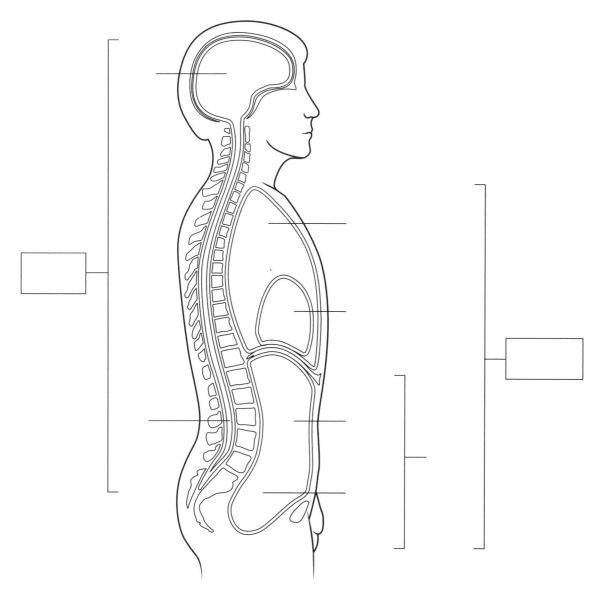

CROSSWORD PUZZLE

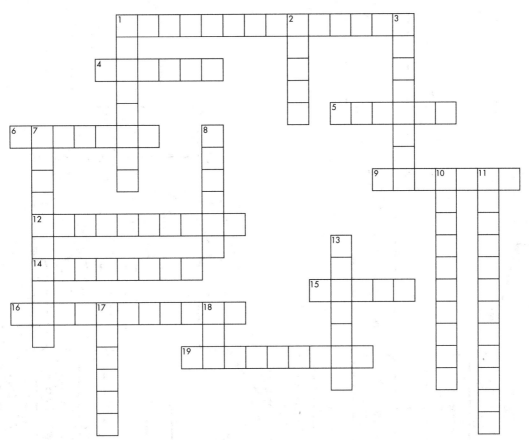

Across

1. body cavity inferior to the diaphragm
4. far from origin
5. face up
6. thigh
9. buttocks
12. standard body position
14. cavity superior to diaphragm
15. face down
16. _____ terms; used to describe anatomy
19. abdominal region surrounding belly button

Down

1. armpit
2. foot
3. neck
7. abdominal region on top of stomach
8. back
10. divides body into superior and inferior sections
11. forearm
13. divides body into anterior and posterior parts
17. wrist
18. brachial

Name _____

CONCEPT MAP

Fill in the empty boxes with an appropriate term using the clues provided.

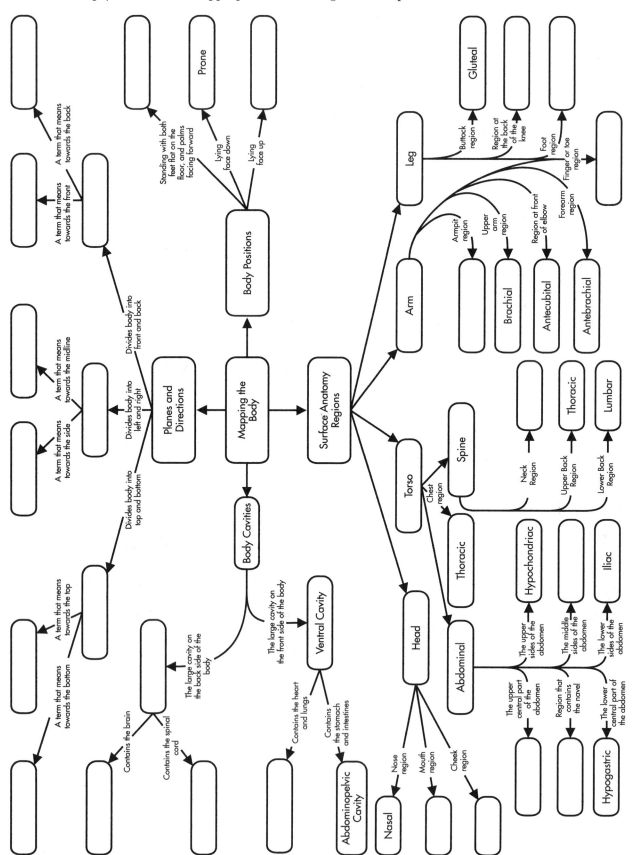

CROSSWORD PUZZLE

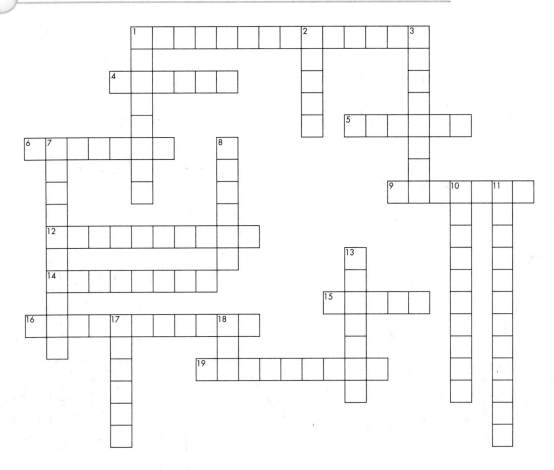

Across

1. body cavity inferior to the diaphragm
4. far from origin
5. face up
6. thigh
9. buttocks
12. standard body position
14. cavity superior to diaphragm
15. face down
16. _____ terms; used to describe anatomy
19. abdominal region surrounding belly button

Down

1. armpit
2. foot
3. neck
7. abdominal region on top of stomach
8. back
10. divides body into superior and inferior sections
11. forearm
13. divides body into anterior and posterior parts
17. wrist
18. brachial

Name _____

CONCEPT MAP

Fill in the empty boxes with an appropriate term using the clues provided.

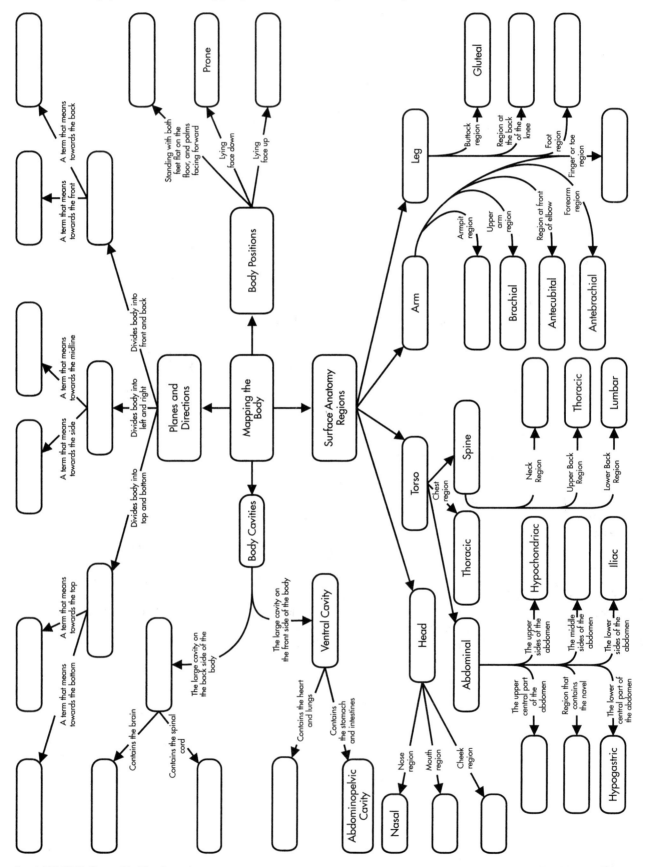

BIOCHEMISTRY: THE BASIC INGREDIENTS OF LIFE

Chapter 3

MEDICAL TERMINOLOGY REVIEW

Define the following terms.

1. Steroid: _____
2. pH: _____
3. Electrolytes: _____
4. Hydrophobic: _____
5. Solution: _____
6. Concentration: _____
7. Biological molecules: _____
8. Glucose: _____
9. Glycogen: _____
10. Metabolism: _____

MULTIPLE CHOICE

Circle the letter of the correct answer.

1. Cellular respiration makes ATP and uses:
   a. glycogen.
   b. glucose.
   c. water.
   d. carbon dioxide.

2. In an enzyme catalyzed reaction, the molecules that bind to enzymes are called:
   a. products.
   b. reactants.
   c. substrates.
   d. proteins.

3. Which of the following is true of enzyme reactions?
   a. Enzymes are not used up
   b. Enzymes are nonspecific
   c. Enzymes are carbohydrates
   d. All of the above

4. Many catabolic reactions are _____ reactions.
   a. dehydration
   b. hydrophobic
   c. hydrolysis
   d. hyperactive

5. Which of the following is a function of proteins?
   a. Structure
   b. Nutrient storage
   c. Communication
   d. All of the above

6. Which of the following is a steroid?
   a. Cholesterol
   b. Ethanol
   c. Preventall
   d. Phospholipid

Copyright © 2020 by Pearson Education, Inc.

7. This is the most hydrophobic molecule known:
   a. phospholipid.
   b. cholesterol.
   c. triglyceride.
   d. wax.

8. Most carbohydrates have this function:
   a. endometriosis.
   b. energy storage.
   c. structure.
   d. waterproofing.

9. How many carbons do simple sugars have?
   a. Four
   b. Ten
   c. Six
   d. Eight

10. A solution is a _____ dissolved in a _____.
    a. solute, solution
    b. solute, solvent
    c. solvent, solute
    d. solution, solute

11. In _____ bonds, electrons are donated.
    a. covalent
    b. polar covalent
    c. ionic
    d. hydrogen

12. A solution with a pH of 8 is:
    a. acidic
    b. neutral
    c. basic
    d. ionic

13. What surround the nucleus in an atom?
    a. Electrons
    b. Protons
    c. Neutrons
    d. Introns

14. These atomic particles are negatively charged:
    a. Positrons
    b. Protons
    c. Neutrons
    d. Electrons

15. This element is needed for formation of hemoglobin:
    a. sodium.
    b. manganese.
    c. calcium.
    d. iron.

16. Atoms that gain or lose electrons are called:
    a. elements.
    b. covalent.
    c. ions.
    d. acids.

17. Molecules that will mix with water are:
    a. hydrophobic.
    b. hydrophilic.
    c. hydrolysis.
    d. hydrogenated.

18. A molecule has several nitrogens in the backbone of the molecule. It is most likely a:
    a. carbohydrate.
    b. lipid.
    c. protein.
    d. nucleic acid.

19. A molecule has two hydrogens and one oxygen for every carbon. What kind of molecule is it?
    a. Carbohydrate
    b. Lipid
    c. Protein
    d. Nucleic acid

20. These molecules have both hydrophobic and hydrophilic portions:
    a. waxes.
    b. phospholipids.
    c. triglycerides.
    d. oils.

21. Ultimately, we need to breathe because:
    a. we need oxygen to make proteins.
    b. we need oxygen to make nucleic acids.
    c. we need oxygen to make carbohydrates.
    d. we need oxygen to make ATP.

22. Which of the following is NOT a biological molecule?
    a. Ethanol
    b. Gasoline
    c. Glucose
    d. DNA

23. What type of molecule is an egg white?
    a. Carbohydrate
    b. Lipid
    c. Protein
    d. Amino Acid

24. A molecule that is made of a phosphate, sugar, and base is a(n):
    a. amino acid.
    b. hydrochloric acid.
    c. nucleic acid.
    d. All of the above

25. Which of the following is a characteristic of enzymes?
    a. Saturation
    b. Specificity
    c. Competition
    d. All of the above

MATCHING EXERCISES

Match each term with the appropriate definition.

Set 1

_____ 1. glucose	a. disaccharide
_____ 2. sucrose	b. steroid
_____ 3. egg-white albumin	c. an electrolyte
_____ 4. RNA	d. monosaccharide
_____ 5. cholesterol	e. an acid
_____ 6. glycogen	f. nucleic acid
_____ 7. Zn	g. high-energy molecule
_____ 8. Na+	h. polysaccharide
_____ 9. HCl	i. protein
_____ 10. ATP	j. a trace element

Set 2

_____ 1. zinc	a. enzyme systems
_____ 2. copper	b. teeth and bones
_____ 3. iron	c. thyroid gland
_____ 4. manganese	d. cellular respiration
_____ 5. iodine	e. hemoglobin
_____ 6. fluorine	f. cell membrane
_____ 7. oxygen	g. CNS, fat metabolism
_____ 8. water	h. genetic code
_____ 9. phospholipids	i. chief biological solvent
_____ 10. DNA	j. amino acid metabolism

Set 3

_____ 1. protein
_____ 2. adenine
_____ 3. polysaccharide
_____ 4. oil
_____ 5. wax
_____ 6. phospholipid
_____ 7. molecule
_____ 8. disaccharide
_____ 9. carbohydrate
_____ 10. enzyme

a. glycerol and fatty acids
b. monosaccharides
c. CH_2O
d. amino acids
e. atoms
f. two monosaccharides
g. fatty acid with alcohol
h. protein with binding site
i. nucleic acid
j. phosphate head and fatty acid tails

Set 4

_____ 1. metabolism
_____ 2. saturation
_____ 3. inhibition
_____ 4. hydrolysis
_____ 5. denaturation
_____ 6. hydrophilic
_____ 7. dehydration synthesis
_____ 8. concentration
_____ 9. biological molecules
_____ 10. steroids

a. amount of solute dissolved in solvent
b. enzyme is blocked
c. can mix with water
d. all the chemical reactions in the body
e. making molecules by removing water
f. adding water to break down molecules
g. include carbohydrates, lipids, proteins, and nucleic acids
h. binding sites are full
i. ringed lipids
j. proteins lose their structure

FILL IN THE BLANK

Fill in the blanks to complete the following statements.

1. Two or more elements joined together form a(n) _____.
2. Elements are usually abbreviated using the _____ of their technical name.
3. A fatty acid that contains a single covalent bond is called _____.
4. Positively charged particles found in the nucleus of an atom are _____.
5. Polar molecules are _____.
6. Ions found in the body are _____.
7. One of the main functions of the _____ system is to regulate electrolyte balance.
8. HCO_3^- is _____ ion.
9. A(n) _____ can release hydrogen ions.
10. A bond with unequal sharing of electrons is a _____ bond.

11. In a solution, the substance doing the dissolving is the _____.
12. Steroids are called "anabolic" because they _____ tissues.
13. Enzymes _____ biological reactions.
14. Only some substances can be carried by enzymes, thus, enzymes are _____.
15. ATP is made in this organelle: _____.
16. The two waste products from cellular respiration are _____ and _____.
17. When ATP gives off energy, it loses a phosphate and becomes _____.
18. Carbon dioxide is a weak _____.
19. Most anabolic reactions are _____ reactions.
20. Negatively charged subatomic particles are _____.
21. A special link called a _____ is found in proteins.
22. Normal saline solution, when mixed with a drug, would be considered a(n) _____.
23. An atom is the smallest recognizable unit of a(n) _____.
24. These molecules may be used for defense, communication, structure, and muscle: _____.
25. Neutral pH is pH _____.

SHORT ANSWER

1. Explain how enzymes work.
   _____
   _____
   _____
   _____

2. List the four classes of biological molecules and their characteristics.
   _____
   _____
   _____
   _____

3. Explain the three types of bonds.

   _____
   _____
   _____
   _____

4. Explain cellular respiration.

   _____
   _____
   _____
   _____

5. Explain metabolism.

   _____
   _____
   _____
   _____

LEARNING ACTIVITIES

1. Research how biochemistry relates to activities in a hospital laboratory.
2. Research various related professional careers in biochemistry.

CROSSWORD PUZZLE

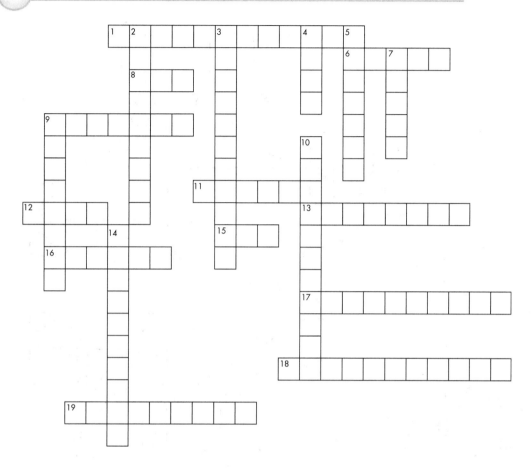

Across

1. has molecular formula CH$_2$O
6. has lots of H and C but little O
8. high energy molecule made during cellular respiration
9. monosaccharide, necessary for cellular respiration
11. dissolved in a solution
12. hydrogen _____ occurs between adjacent water molecules
13. when atoms share electrons
15. charged atom or molecule
16. speeds up rates of biological reactions
17. breaking down large molecules
18. water loving
19. the building block of protein (2 words)

Down

2. building large molecules out of small ones
3. will not mix with water
4. smallest recognizable unit of an element
5. smallest unit of specific type of matter
7. charged
9. polysaccharide
10. only certain molecules can fit in a binding site
14. adding water to split molecules

Name _____

CONCEPT MAP

Fill in the empty boxes with an appropriate term using the clues provided.

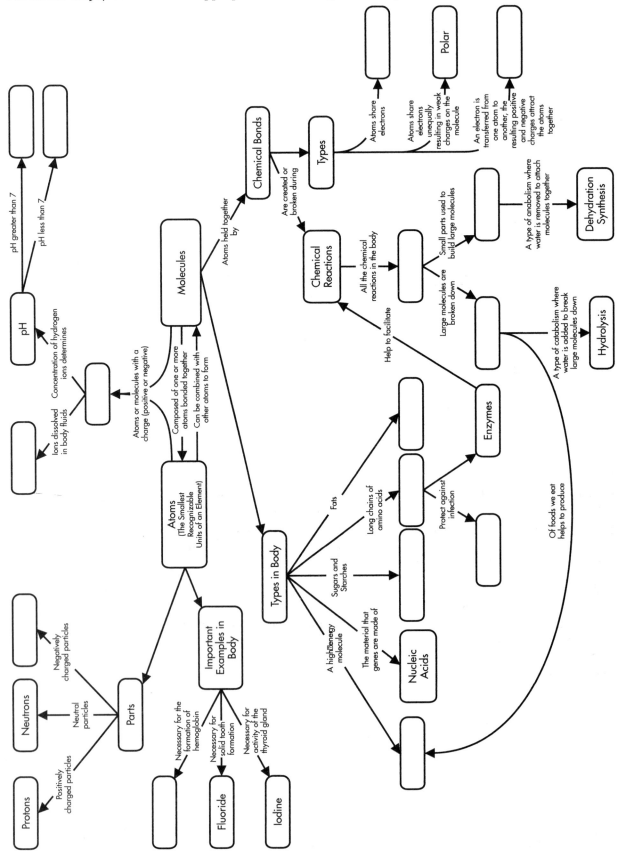

THE CELLS: THE RAW MATERIALS AND BUILDING BLOCKS

Chapter 4

MEDICAL TERMINOLOGY REVIEW

Define the following terms.

1. Nucleus: _____
2. Cellular respiration: _____
3. Cancer: _____
4. Semipermeable: _____
5. Antibiotic: _____
6. Mitosis: _____
7. Organelle: _____
8. Pathogen: _____
9. Virus: _____
10. Bacteria: _____

MULTIPLE CHOICE

Circle the letter of the correct answer.

1. The movement of water across a semipermeable membrane is called:
   a. diffusion.
   b. osmosis.
   c. phagocytosis.
   d. exocytosis.

2. Where is DNA synthesized?
   a. Endoplasmic reticulum
   b. Lysosomes
   c. Golgi apparatus
   d. Nucleus

3. Which mechanism uses ATP?
   a. exocytosis.
   b. pinocytosis.
   c. endocytosis.
   d. All of the above

4. The microorganism that causes herpes is a:
   a. bacterium.
   b. protozoan.
   c. virus.
   d. fungus.

5. A sperm cell propels itself with a single whiplike structure. This type of structure is called a:
   a. flagellum.
   b. cilium.
   c. tinea cordae.
   d. cordae equina.

Copyright © 2020 by Pearson Education, Inc.

6. Containers A and B are separated by a semipermeable membrane. The solute concentration is 6 mg/ml in container A and 2 mg/ml in container B. In what direction will *osmosis* take place?
   a. B to A
   b. No movement can take place
   c. A to B
   d. From A to B first and then from B to A for stability

7. What process occurs across the walls of small blood vessels, pushing both water and dissolved nutrients into the tissues of the body?
   a. Osmosis
   b. Diffusion
   c. Filtration
   d. Hemolysis

8. In what part of the nucleus are instructions for protein synthesis stored?
   a. RNA
   b. DNA
   c. Nucleolus
   d. Lysosome

9. When a membrane allows only certain substances in and out, the membrane is said to be:
   a. semipermeable.
   b. selectively permeable.
   c. impermeable.
   d. a and b.

10. Which molecule keeps hydrophilic molecules from easily crossing cell membranes?
    a. Protein
    b. Carbohydrates
    c. Phospholipids
    d. Cholesterol

11. The inner membrane of the trachea moves phlegm upward in a wavelike motion with its microscopic hairlike projections. These types of structures are called:
    a. flagella.
    b. cilia.
    c. endoplasmic reticula.
    d. receptors.

12. This type of cellular transport moves substances against the concentration gradient:
    a. diffusion.
    b. filtration.
    c. active pump.
    d. osmosis.

13. Glucose needs to be ushered into the cells using:
    a. facilitated diffusion.
    b. phagocytosis.
    c. pinocytosis.
    d. exocytosis.

14. Which of the following is NOT a characteristic of carriers?
    a. Saturation
    b. Prohibition
    c. Inhibition
    d. Competition

15. Which of the following is a type of transport through a cell membrane with or along the concentration gradient?
    a. Active transport pumps
    b. Diffusion
    c. Phagocytosis
    d. Exocytosis

16. The microorganism that causes athlete's foot is a:
    a. bacterium.
    b. virus.
    c. fungus.
    d. protozoan.

17. Postural muscles, such as muscles of the neck, are in constant need of energy. Therefore, these muscle cells contain and maintain higher quantities of what type of organelles than do cells not requiring high-energy stores?
    a. Mitochondria
    b. Nucleus
    c. Ribosomes
    d. Endoplasmic reticulum

18. This part of the cell cycle is cell division:
    a. mitosis.
    b. interphase.
    c. cytokinesis.
    d. metaphase.

19. A pathogen is a(n):
    a. organism that produces disease.
    b. host for viruses.
    c. cellular receptor.
    d. internal method of transport.

20. This type of cell has no true nucleus or nuclear membrane:
    a. eukaryotic.
    b. prokaryotic.
    c. gamete.
    d. virus.

21. There are two classes of tumors. The type that will spread is called:
    a. malignant.
    b. sigma.
    c. bacteria.
    d. benign.

22. Which of the following is a waste product from cellular respiration that must be removed from the body?
    a. Adenosine triphosphate
    b. Water
    c. Carbon dioxide
    d. Glucose

23. An activated canister of tear gas is thrown into a room. Soon the gas has spread wall to wall and floor to ceiling. This movement of the gas is an example of:
    a. diffusion.
    b. endocytosis.
    c. osmosis.
    d. pinocytosis.

24. When a cancerous tumor breaks off and travels to other parts of the body, it is said be:
    a. thrombosized.
    b. embolized.
    c. metastasized.
    d. dormant.

25. Candidiasis is common in some people who have AIDS. Candidiasis is result of what type of infection?
    a. Protozoan
    b. Fungal
    c. Viral
    d. Bacterial

MATCHING EXERCISES

Match each term with the appropriate definition.

Set 1

_____ 1. passive
_____ 2. active
_____ 3. diffusion
_____ 4. filtration
_____ 5. pinocytosis
_____ 6. exocytosis
_____ 7. endocytosis
_____ 8. phagocytosis
_____ 9. active transport pumps
_____ 10. osmosis

a. pressure is applied to force water and dissolved material across a membrane
b. intake of liquid and food by cells by engulfing
c. movement of substances from higher concentration to lower concentration
d. general term for a type of transport that requires energy
e. movement of water from areas of low concentration of solute to areas that have high concentration of solute
f. how a cell transports things out of itself using a vesicle
g. general term for a type of transport that requires no energy
h. "pushing" more into the cell using ATP as energy
i. specifically, the intake of liquid into cells by engulfing
j. specifically, the intake of solid particles into cells by engulfing

Set 2

____ 1. cell membrane
____ 2. nucleolus
____ 3. ribosome
____ 4. lysosome
____ 5. mitochondria
____ 6. endoplasmic reticulum
____ 7. Golgi apparatus
____ 8. centrioles
____ 9. chromatids
____ 10. cytoplasm

a. a series of transport channels in the cell, having two distinct forms
b. where RNA is synthesized
c. produces ATP
d. containing powerful enzymes
e. contains DNA
f. gel-like substance in which the cellular organelles float
g. plays a critical role in cell division
h. attaches to rough ER and produces protein
i. surrounds the cells and allows certain substances in and out
j. puts proteins into vesicles

Set 3

____ 1. bacteria
____ 2. malaria
____ 3. prion
____ 4. virus
____ 5. pathogenic
____ 6. capsid
____ 7. athlete's foot
____ 8. shingles
____ 9. fungus
____ 10. protozoa

a. microorganism that contributes to the normal flora of the body; can be pathogenic or nonpathogenic
b. the coat that surrounds the genetic material of a virus
c. recurrence of chicken pox
d. an adjective used when an organism is said to produce disease
e. microorganism that cannot reproduce or eat by itself; needs a host
f. a disease caused by a protozoa living inside mosquitoes
g. general term for one-celled, animal-like organisms responsible for many tropical disease transmitted through consumption of unclean water
h. plantlike organism that can be either one-celled or multicelled
i. a causative agent in certain brain diseases
j. a common fungal infection of the skin

Set 4

____ 1. eukaryote
____ 2. prokaryote
____ 3. interphase
____ 4. metastasis
____ 5. cytokinesis
____ 6. mitosis
____ 7. prophase
____ 8. metaphase
____ 9. anaphase
____ 10. telophase

a. nucleus disappears; spindle forms
b. spread of cancer cells
c. chromosomes line up in center of cell
d. cell with nucleus and organelles
e. division of cytoplasm and organelles
f. cell without nucleus and organelles
g. chromosomes pull away
h. time during which cell is not dividing
i. spindle disappears, chromosomes are far apart
j. nuclear division

FILL IN THE BLANK

Fill in the blanks to complete the following statements.

1. The type of transport demonstrated by oxygen being transported from the lungs to the blood is _____.
2. When a cell surrounds a solid particle forming a vesicle and pulls it into the cells, this transport is called _____.
3. ATP stands for _____.
4. The situation in which more potassium is pulled into the cell despite being at a higher concentration inside the cell is called _____.
5. The blueprint of the cell is contained in genetic material called _____.
6. One of the reasons that smoking is so dangerous is that it paralyzes _____, often leading to chronic lung disorders.
7. The microorganism that is not killed by antibiotics is a _____.
8. Certain bacteria in the intestine actually help synthesize vitamin _____.
9. Fungi can spread through the release of _____.
10. In a solution, the substance that is dissolved in water is referred to as the _____.
11. The structural difference between ATP and ADP is the number of _____ groups.
12. The type of microorganism that makes up the normal flora of the human body is _____.
13. The division of the cytoplasm and organelles is called _____.
14. The smallest functional unit of the body is the _____.
15. A disease caused by a protozoan carried within the body of a mosquito is _____.
16. The treatment and course of any infection is determined by the _____ involved.
17. These organelles, _____, contain powerful digestive enzymes.
18. Glucose must get into cells so they can make _____, a higher energy molecule necessary for cell metabolism.
19. These biological molecules often act as carriers: _____.
20. These organelles, _____, are more common in tissues that have high-energy demands.

21. _____ is defined by the uncontrolled growth and spread of cells.
22. Besides glucose, what molecule is required for cells to perform cellular respiration? _____
23. In mitosis, the nucleus disappears during _____.
24. The spread of cancerous cells is called _____.
25. _____ should never be a treatment for a viral infection.

SHORT ANSWER

1. What is the function of the cell membrane?

2. Why don't antibiotics kill viruses?

3. List and briefly describe the phases of mitosis.

4. What is the difference between passive and active transport?

5. Explain the relationship between ATP, ADP, and energy.

LEARNING ACTIVITIES

1. Using the internet as a source, list as many organelles and their disorders as you can.
2. Play "Cell Biology Five Questions." One student selects an organelle or a term and the other students try to guess the organelle by asking questions. Can you get it in 5 questions?
3. There are several websites that offer virtual tours of cells. Take a virtual tour. For each organelle, write down one new fact that you learned. Share your facts with other students in the class until you have generated a list of interesting facts for each organelle.

LABELING ACTIVITY

Label the parts of the cell. Use Figure 4–1 of your textbook as a guide.

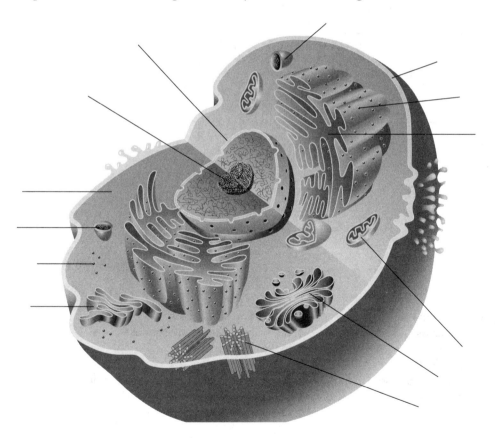

CROSSWORD PUZZLE

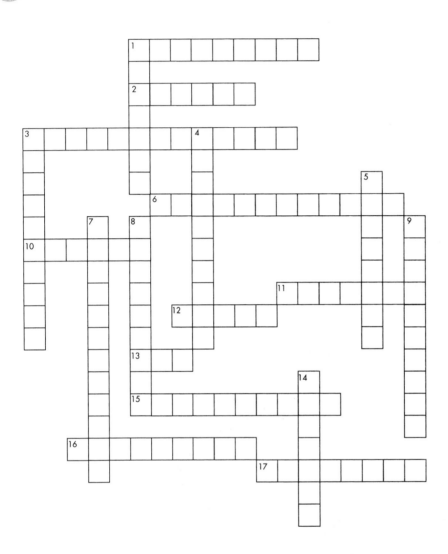

Across
1. make ribosomes
2. cells reproducing out of control
3. only some substances can cross
6. cell engulfing solid particles
10. _____ transport uses ATP
11. broken down during cellular respiration
12. hijacks cell in order to reproduce
13. high energy molecule
15. substance leaves cell in a vesicle
16. movement of substance from high to low concentration
17. vesicle containing powerful enzymes (2 words)

Down
1. contains genetic information for cell
3. all binding sites full
4. cell with nucleus and organelles
5. makes protein
7. makes ATP
8. chromosomes line up in center of cell
9. cell is not dividing
14. cell division of eukaryotic cells

Name _____

CONCEPT MAP

Fill in the empty boxes with an appropriate term using the clues provided.

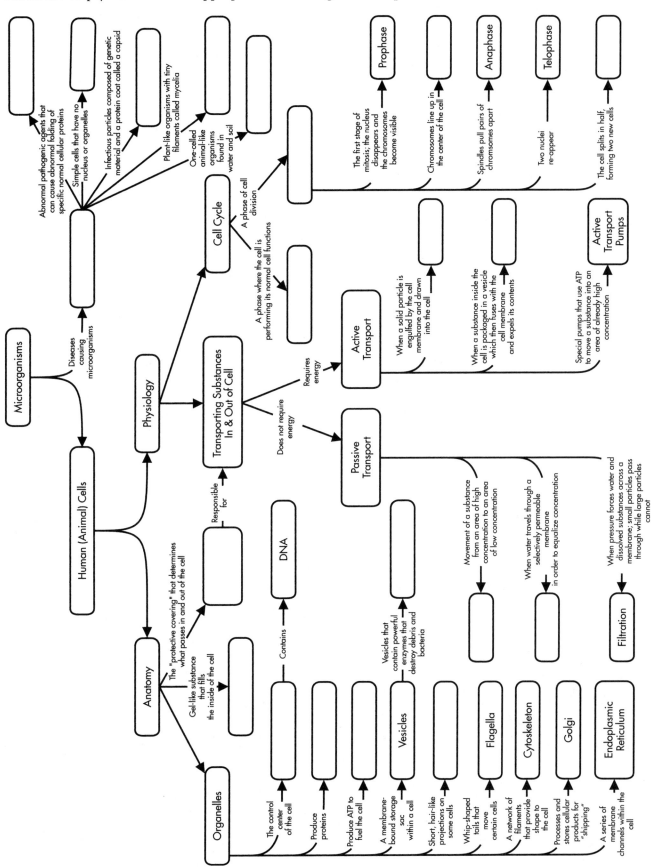

TISSUES AND SYSTEMS: THE INSIDE STORY

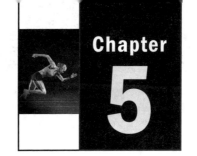

MEDICAL TERMINOLOGY

Define the following terms.
1. Serous: _____
2. Mucous: _____
3. Synovial: _____
4. Stratified: _____
5. Striated: _____
6. Matrix: _____
7. Tissue: _____
8. Organ: _____
9. System: _____
10. Vital: _____

MULTIPLE CHOICE

Circle the letter of the correct answer.

1. When an epithelial tissue is single-layered and made of flat, scale-like cells, what is it called?
   a. Simple scalular
   b. Simple cuboidal
   c. Simple squamous
   d. Simple columnar

2. This type of tissue supports structures and stores nutrients:
   a. epithelial.
   b. connective.
   c. nervous.
   d. muscular.

3. When an epithelial tissue is multiple-layered and made of cells that are taller than they are wide, what are they called?
   a. Stratified columnar
   b. Striated columnar
   c. Stratus columnalis
   d. Strafed columns

4. What is the clinical term for fat?
   a. Synovial tissue
   b. Areolar tissue
   c. Adipose tissue
   d. Cartilaginous tissue

5. What is the function of a neuron?
   a. Conductor of information
   b. Producer of hormone
   c. Protection and support
   d. Storage of fat and protein

6. Which of the following epithelial tissues can be found in the outermost layer of skin?
   a. Stratified cuboidal
   b. Striated scalular
   c. Stratified squamous
   d. Simple squamous

7. Which of the following is a characteristic of epithelial tissue?
   a. Has extensive extracellular matrix
   b. Cells come in a variety of shapes
   c. No obvious top or bottom surface
   d. All are characteristics of epithelial tissue

8. Blood and lymph are considered to be:
   a. synovial tissue.
   b. connective tissue.
   c. serous tissue.
   d. mucous tissue.

9. The membrane that lines cavities that open to the exterior, such as the mouth and the reproductive and respiratory tracts, is called:
   a. mucous membrane.
   b. serous membrane.
   c. visceral membrane.
   d. cutaneous membrane.

10. The visceral layer of a serous membrane:
    a. lines the inside of the skull.
    b. wraps around the individual organs.
    c. holds neurons together.
    d. lines the body cavities.

11. Which of the following is true about the internal structure of skeletal muscle cells?
    a. It is multinucleate.
    b. It contains lacunae.
    c. It has no nucleus.
    d. It has no organelles.

12. Which tissue regenerates easily?
    a. Bone
    b. Cartilage
    c. Nervous
    d. Cardiac

13. Because conscious effort and thought for movement are involved, skeletal muscles are also called:
    a. voluntary muscles.
    b. premeditated muscles.
    c. deliberate muscles.
    d. intentional muscle.

14. Each organ is a group of several different kinds of:
    a. regions.
    b. systems.
    c. muscles.
    d. tissues.

15. Because they are not controlled by conscious thought, cardiac and smooth muscle tissues are considered what kind of muscles?
    a. Habitual
    b. Spontaneous
    c. Involuntary
    d. Instinctive

16. Which of these organs are paired?
    a. Spleens
    b. Kidneys
    c. Livers
    d. Urinary bladders

17. Due to its microscopic appearance in comparison with the skeletal muscle, visceral muscle is called:
    a. little Swiss.
    b. smooth.
    c. rough.
    d. spongy.

18. Which part of the neuron transmits impulses away from the cell body?
    a. Dendrite
    b. Soma
    c. Meninges
    d. Axon

19. The function of hormones is to:
    a. regulate metabolic processes.
    b. regulate fluid balance.
    c. regulate rate of growth and reproduction.
    d. All of the above

20. Where is visceral muscle found in the body?
    a. Digestive system
    b. Cardiovascular system
    c. Urinary system
    d. All of the above

21. Which organ(s) listed is/are considered vital organs?
    a. Gallbladder
    b. Appendix
    c. Brain
    d. All of the above

22. Which body system regulates calcium levels?
    a. Endocrine
    b. Digestive
    c. Lymphatic
    d. Skeletal

23. Graves' disease is caused by immune attack on the thyroid. What body system is involved in this disorder?
    a. Endocrine
    b. Nervous
    c. Cardiovascular
    d. Skeletal

24. These cells are undifferentiated or unspecialized:
    a. osteocytes.
    b. chondrocytes.
    c. stem.
    d. neurons.

25. Which is the correct order of the steps in wound healing?
    a. Inflammation, organization, remodeling
    b. Inflammation, clotting, organization, regeneration (or scarring)
    c. Clotting, fibrosis, regeneration
    d. Fibrosis, regeneration, inflammation, clotting

MATCHING EXERCISES

Match each term with the appropriate definition.

Set 1

1. nervous tissue
2. muscle tissue
3. connective tissue
4. epithelial tissue
5. striated
6. transitional
7. serous
8. meninges
9. cutaneous
10. synovial

a. specifically, the *membrane* that covers the spinal cord and brain
b. tissue that holds things together and provides structure
c. appearance of skeletal muscles
d. has the ability to shorten itself; provides movement by and in our bodies
e. multiple layers of epithelial tissue that can expand and contract
f. found in the space between joints; produces a slippery fluid
g. membrane that covers organs and lines cavities
h. communication; rapid messenger of information
i. commonly known as the skin
j. the tissue type that covers the body and its parts

Set 2

_____ 1. lymphatic system
_____ 2. endocrine system
_____ 3. nervous system
_____ 4. female reproductive system
_____ 5. male reproductive system
_____ 6. digestive system
_____ 7. respiratory system
_____ 8. integumentary system
_____ 9. cardiovascular system
_____ 10. muscular system

a. supports and sustains structure; framework of body
b. movement; controls the diameter of blood vessels
c. surface protection from harmful environmental invaders
d. produces ova and houses the growing fetus
e. communication and control through the release of chemical substances
f. produces red blood cells
g. chemically and mechanically breaks down food for use by the body
h. communication; transmission of impulses
i. transports water, oxygen, and nutrients toward and away from the cells of the body
j. produces sperm
k. maintains proper fluid balance in the body; helps fight disease
l. supplies fresh oxygen for the bloodstream

Set 3

_____ 1. both pancreas and testes
_____ 2. both vas deferens and penis
_____ 3. tonsils and lymph vessels
_____ 4. heart and veins
_____ 5. small intestine and gallbladder
_____ 6. kidneys
_____ 7. sweat and oil glands
_____ 8. brain and spinal cord
_____ 9. trachea and bronchus
_____ 10. uterus and fallopian tubes

a. belong to the system that produces sperm
b. belong to the system that produces urine
c. belong to the system that digests and eliminates food
d. belong to the system that contains sensory and motor neurons
e. belong to the system that produces hormones
f. belong to the system that allows us to flex and extend bones at movable joints
g. belong to the system that covers and protects the body
h. belong to the system that allows for the union of the sperm and ova
i. belong to the system that eliminates carbon dioxide from the body
j. belong to the system that includes blood
k. belong to the system that cleans up excess fluid and fights infections

Set 4

____ 1. areolar tissue
____ 2. dense regular connective tissue
____ 3. bone
____ 4. blood
____ 5. adipose tissue
____ 6. cartilage
____ 7. skeletal muscle
____ 8. cardiac muscle
____ 9. stratified columnar epithelium
____ 10. transitional epithelium

a. striated, cylindrical multinucleate
b. cells in lacunae; mineral matrix
c. multiple layers, tall, thin cells
d. weblike general purpose connective tissue
e. cells in liquid matrix
f. stretchy cells of various shapes
g. striated, branched, uninucleate, connected
h. cells in lacunae, gel-like matrix
i. cells full of lipids
j. packed with parallel collagen fibers

FILL IN THE BLANK

Fill in the blanks to complete the following statements.

1. Both visceral and parietal membranes are part of _____ membranes.
2. The organ with which the cardiac muscle is associated is called the _____.
3. A neuron is one type of nerve cell; the other type of nerve cell is called _____.
4. The testes belong to the reproductive and the _____ systems.
5. The pancreas belongs to the endocrine and the _____ systems.
6. Hormones circulate through the _____ system.
7. Sight, hearing, touch, taste, and smell belong to the _____ system.
8. The second name of an epithelial tissue is determined by _____ of its cells.
9. _____ are the support cells in nervous tissue.
10. Pseudostratified _____ tissues line the lower part of the digestive tract.
11. Storing nutrients is a function of _____ tissue.
12. When muscles are striped in appearance, they are said to be _____.
13. The membrane that lines joints produces a fluid that reduces friction called _____.
14. Tendons and ligaments are composed of dense _____ tissue.
15. The spleen belongs to the _____ system.
16. Diabetes may be related to tissue damage because the disease inhibits _____.

17. Patients who are obese have excess _____ tissue.
18. If your pleura are inflamed, where is the pain? _____
19. _____ tissue does not regenerate.
20. Nonliving material surrounding cells is called _____.
21. You are given the following tissue to examine: It has clusters of cells in tiny holes, a matrix like Jell-O, and fibers. What kind of tissue is it? _____
22. The most important difference between epithelium and connective tissue is that connective tissue has a _____.
23. Medicine that is researching the use of stem cells to treat disease is called _____.
24. You are given the following tissue to examine: It is a sheet of tightly packed cells and nothing else. What type of tissue is it? _____
25. A cell that has the ability to differentiate into various cell types is called _____.

SHORT ANSWER

1. List and describe the four main types of tissues.

2. Differentiate the three main types of muscle tissue.

3. Explain tissue repair.

4. Describe the structure and function of a serous membrane.

5. Compare the similarities of the endocrine and the nervous systems.

_____
_____
_____
_____

LEARNING ACTIVITIES

1. For each system, list as many organs as you can without looking.
2. Make a deck of cards. For each pair of cards, write the name of an organ on one card and the name of the system on the other card. Play "Concentration," matching organs with their correct system.
3. Play "Tissue Anatomical Illustrator." One student draws a type of tissue. Other students guess the type of tissue based on cell shape and other physical characteristics.
4. Write a decision tree (dichotomous key) for the tissues to practice telling them apart. For each characteristic, answer yes or no for the tissue you are describing. Each decision will eliminate one type of tissue until you have arrived at the right identification by process of elimination. If you search for "dichotomous key to tissues," you will find several examples on the internet. Once you have written the key, try using it to identify slides.
5. There are many different tissue disorders not discussed in this book. Use the internet to research disorders for one particular type of tissue.

LABELING ACTIVITY

Label each type of tissue. Use Figure 5–1 of your textbook as a guide.

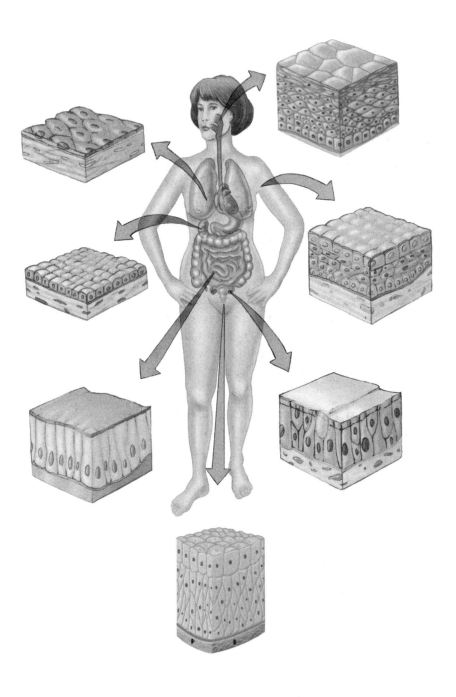

CROSSWORD PUZZLE

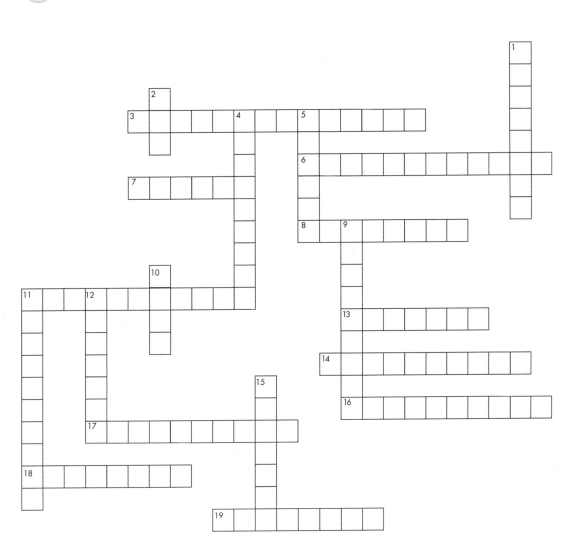

Across

3. the heart is part of the _____ system
6. wound is repaired by original tissue
7. this system fights infection
8. the _____ system makes red blood cells
11. cartilage cell
13. muscle with connections between cells
14. cell that repairs damaged tissue
16. _____ tissue has no extracellular matrix
17. tissue with more than one layer of cells
18. the _____ layer of the pericardium covers the heart surface
19. skeletal muscle is _____ muscle

Down

1. plate-like cells
2. common name for adipose tissue
4. mature bone cell
5. double layered membrane
9. this system controls the body by releasing hormones
10. cells in mineral matrix
11. tissue with extracellular matrix
12. this system contains the brain, spinal cord, nerves
15. web-like support tissue

Name _____

CONCEPT MAP

Fill in the empty boxes with an appropriate term using the clues provided.

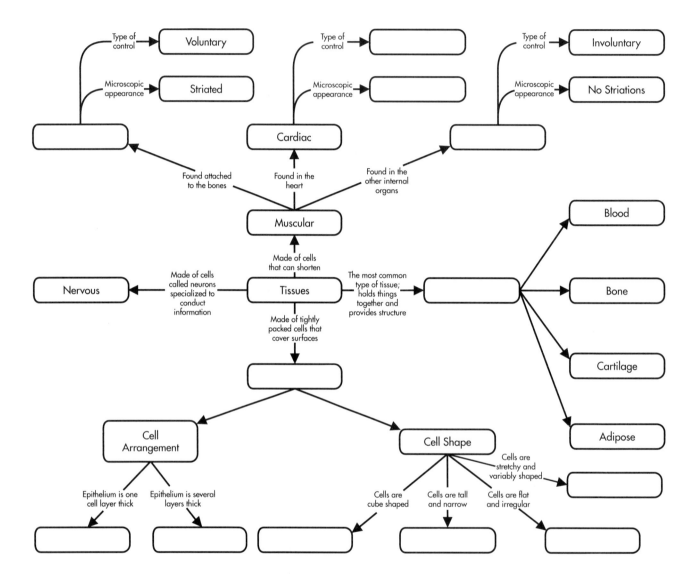

Name _____

CONCEPT MAP

Fill in the empty boxes with an appropriate term using the clues provided.

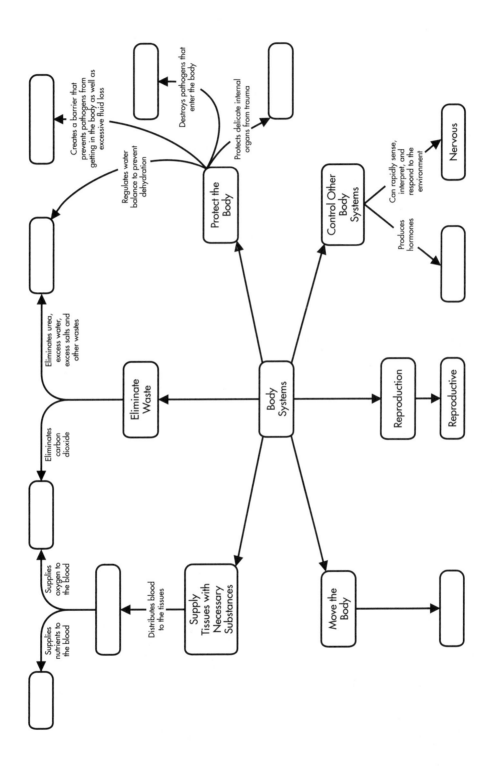

THE SKELETAL SYSTEM: THE FRAMEWORK

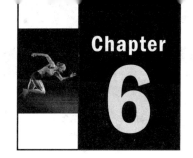

Chapter 6

MEDICAL TERMINOLOGY REVIEW

Define the following terms.

1. Osteoporosis: _____
2. Arthritis: _____
3. Ossification: _____
4. Osteon: _____
5. Articulation: _____
6. Ligament: _____
7. Tendon: _____
8. Reduction: _____
9. Sternum: _____
10. Comminuted fracture: _____

MULTIPLE CHOICE

Circle the letter of the correct answer.

1. What is a fracture that breaks the skin called?
   a. Simple fracture
   b. Closed fracture
   c. Compound fracture
   d. Greenstick

2. Which is the second stage in bone repair?
   a. Remodeling
   b. Soft callus formation
   c. Hematoma formation and inflammation
   d. Bony callus formation

3. During endochondral ossification, osteoblasts invade the center of the diaphysis, forming the:
   a. primary ossification center.
   b. secondary ossification center.
   c. medullary cavity.
   d. endosteal cavity.

4. Which of the following allows the human body to absorb ingested calcium from the digestive tract?
   a. Iron
   b. Vitamin B
   c. Vitamin D
   d. Phosphorus

5. Which of the following "vices," according to the textbook, decreases bone mass?
   a. Caffeine: coffee or cola
   b. Tobacco: cigarette smoking
   c. Bourbon: overindulgence in the spirits
   d. Chocolate: constantly feeding a candy craving
   e. a and b
   f. a, b, c, d

6. Before a bone can heal, what must be done to it to make sure the ends of the bone are touching?
   a. Immobilize it.
   b. Reduce it.
   c. Repair it.
   d. Rebreak it.

7. What is the function of osteoblasts?
   a. Tear down bone
   b. Build new bone
   c. Absorb calcium from the gut
   d. Stimulate calcium retention in the kidneys

8. Where are osteoprogenitor cells found?
   a. Periosteum
   b. Spleen
   c. Bone marrow
   d. Thymus

9. The primary component of the skeleton is:
   a. synovial fluid.
   b. cartilage.
   c. bone.
   d. ligament.

10. The phalanges and ulna are examples of what type of bone?
    a. Irregularly shaped
    b. Long
    c. Short
    d. Flat

11. The mandible and cervical vertebrae are examples of what type of bone?
    a. Irregularly shaped
    b. Long
    c. Short
    d. Flat

12. Most fibrous joints are:
    a. joined by cartilage.
    b. freely moving.
    c. joined by a joint cavity.
    d. slightly movable.

13. The expanded ends of long bones are called:
    a. epimysia.
    b. epicondyles.
    c. epiphyses.
    d. epiosteum.

14. What substance is housed in spongy bone, yet absent in the medullary cavity?
    a. Progenitor cells
    b. Red bone marrow
    c. Yellow bone marrow
    d. Digestive enzymes

15. What type of bony tissue makes up the adult diaphysis?
    a. Cancellous bone
    b. Spongy bone
    c. Cartilage
    d. Compact bone

16. Mature bone cells are clinically called:
    a. osteocytes.
    b. osteoblasts.
    c. osteoprogenitor.
    d. osteoclasts.

17. Mature bone cells are housed in tiny holes known as:
    a. lacunae.
    b. lamellae.
    c. perforating canals.
    d. central canals.

18. Shaking the head in an aggressive gesture of "no" is employing:
    a. adduction/abduction.
    b. rotation.
    c. flexion/extension.
    d. supination/pronation.

19. Connective tissue that attaches bone to bone is called:
    a. ligament.
    b. cartilage.
    c. tendon.
    d. fascia.

20. Moving the joints of the ankle and foot so that the sole of the foot is facing down is called:
    a. pronation.
    b. eversion.
    c. hyperadduction.
    d. plantar flexion.

21. Which of the following bones belong to the axial skeleton?
    a. Clavicle
    b. Scapula
    c. Hyoid
    d. Tarsal

22. Which of the following bones belong to the appendicular skeleton?
    a. Ribs
    b. Sternum
    c. Femur
    d. Sacrum

23. The tip of the sternum is called the:
    a. xyphoid.
    b. hyoid.
    c. condyloid.
    d. patella.

24. The vertebral column has how many vertebrae in the sacral, cervical, lumbar, and thoracic regions?
    a. 7, 12, 5, 5
    b. 3–4, 12, 5, 5
    c. 5, 7, 5, 12
    d. 1–4, 7, 12, 5

25. Besides depression and elevation, which of the following is also an action of the human mandible?
    a. Protraction and retraction
    b. Supination and pronation
    c. Inversion and eversion
    d. Flexion and extension

MATCHING EXERCISES

Match each term with the appropriate definition.

Set 1

1. true ribs
2. shoulder blade
3. upper arm bone
4. fingers and toes
5. thigh bone
6. lower leg bone
7. forearm bone
8. wrist bones
9. ankle bones
10. foot bones

a. clavicle
b. metatarsals
c. scapula
d. radius
e. femur
f. vertebrocostal
g. fibula
h. tarsals
i. phalanges
j. humerus
k. carpals
l. metacarpals
m. vertebrosternal

Set 2

_____ 1. ellipsoidal
_____ 2. synovial
_____ 3. ball and socket
_____ 4. gliding
_____ 5. saddle
_____ 6. pivot
_____ 7. suture
_____ 8. cartilaginous
_____ 9. fibrous
_____ 10. hinge

a. neck and forearm; rotates
b. found at the pubic symphysis and joins the ribs to the sternum
c. hips and shoulder; multiple movement
d. knees and elbows; allows for flexion and extension
e. found on the cranium; sutures
f. base of the thumb; multiple movement including opposition
g. fluid in a joint cavity
h. joints with very short connective tissue strands; between bones of skull
i. found between the carpals and between the tarsals
j. found between wrist bones and the forearm bones; allows biaxial movement

Set 3

_____ 1. diaphysis
_____ 2. facet
_____ 3. tubercle
_____ 4. fossa
_____ 5. meatus
_____ 6. sinus
_____ 7. crest
_____ 8. head
_____ 9. foramen
_____ 10. spine

a. a tube or tunnel-like passageway through a bone
b. a nontubular passageway through a bone for ligament, nerves, and blood vessels
c. a small flattened area
d. the shaft of the bone
e. a knoblike projection
f. a sharp pointed projection
g. a hollow area; space within a bone
h. an articulating end of a bone that is rounded
i. a narrow ridge
j. shallow depression

Set 4

_____ 1. flexion
_____ 2. extension
_____ 3. rotation
_____ 4. circumduction
_____ 5. abduction
_____ 6. adduction
_____ 7. protraction
_____ 8. retraction
_____ 9. elevation
_____ 10. depression

a. decrease joint angle
b. move toward anterior
c. move toward center of body
d. spin on axis
e. move toward inferior
f. increase joint angle
g. move away from center of body
h. move toward posterior
i. move toward superior
j. end of bone moves in circle

FILL IN THE BLANK

Fill in the blanks to complete the following statements.

1. The medical condition called _____ is a degenerative disorder characterized by a decrease in bone density.
2. Cleft palate and club foot are examples of _____ disorders.
3. Secondary curvatures of the spine are found in the _____ and _____ vertebral regions.
4. According to your text, osteoclasts arise from _____.
5. If you move the joint of the ankle and foot so that you are standing on the ball of the foot, you have then _____ the foot.
6. When a joint is straightened or merely moved so that the angle between the individual bones has increased, the movement is termed _____.
7. The bone called the _____ is commonly known as the lower jaw.
8. During CPR chest compressions, the part called the _____ of the sternum takes the brunt of the compressive force.
9. Ribs 8, 9, and 10 can be clinically called _____, or commonly called false ribs.
10. Similar to the elbow joint, interphalangeal joints are _____ joints.
11. In the creation of the skeletal bones, when shaped cartilage is replaced by osseous tissue, this process is known as _____.
12. Where bursitis is inflammation of a bursa, inflammation of the joint is called _____.
13. The human skeleton has _____ bones.
14. Falling off his skateboard, Hugh experienced a _____ fracture due to the bones of his forearm being crushed to the point of splintering.
15. Specialized cells called _____ are needed to tear down bone.
16. The last step in bone repair is _____.
17. The canals that run from osteon to osteon are known as _____ canals.
18. Most of your bones are made of _____ prior to embryonic week 8.
19. Bone matrix is made mainly of two minerals: _____ and _____.

20. _____ bone is composed of cylinders known as osteons.
21. Falling off his skateboard, Hugh experienced a fracture of the bones of his forearm. These bones, the _____ and the _____ were injured.
22. Osteoporosis may in part be due to excessive activity of these cells: _____.
23. _____ in the skull are connective joints that help absorb shock following a blow to the head.
24. Spongy bone is composed mainly of strips of bone known as _____.
25. A medullary cavity is in the center of a long bone. _____ is in the center of short, flat, and irregular bones.

SHORT ANSWER

1. What are four functions of the skeleton?

2. Compare and contrast the four types of bones.

3. What are the functions of the periosteum?

4. Discuss the difference between a ligament and a tendon.

5. Explain ossification.

_____
_____
_____
_____

LEARNING ACTIVITIES

1. Get a cutout of a skeleton—perhaps a Halloween decoration. How many bones can you name?
2. Take a survey of the students in the class or your friends and the members of your family. How many have had bone and or joint injuries? What was the treatment? Make a table of types of injuries and treatments.
3. Buy an inexpensive plastic skeleton from a hobby shop or card store. Take it apart. Can you put it back together?
4. Get into pairs and demonstrate joint movements. Can you tell which is which? See who can make the correct movement when "ordered" to do it by another student.
5. For each joint, figure out which movements it can make. Does the list make sense given the structure of the joint?

LABELING ACTIVITY

Label and color the parts of the bone indicated here. Use Figure 6–2 from your textbook as a guide.

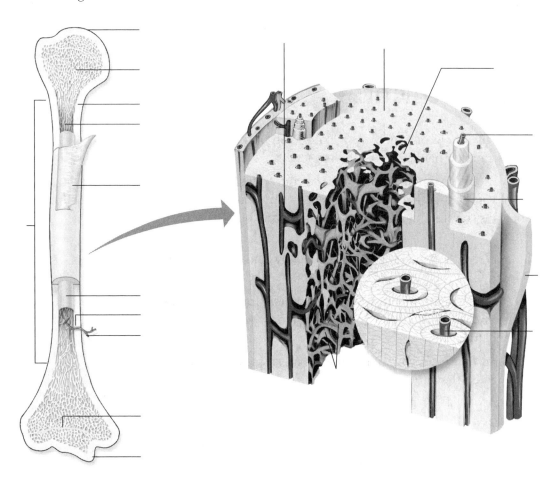

CROSSWORD PUZZLE

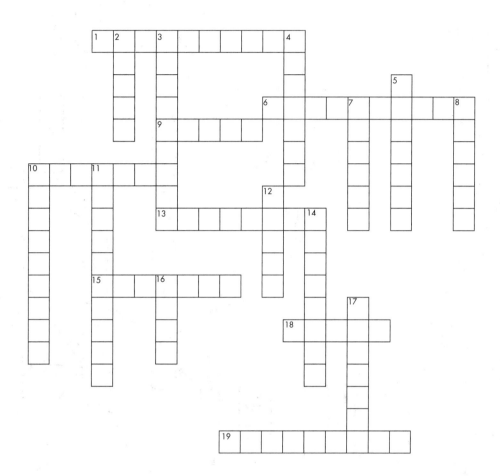

Across

1. cell which makes bone
6. cell which tears down bone
9. a joint which only flexes and extends
10. wrist bones
13. membrane lining freely moving joints
15. breastbone
18. thigh bone
19. shaft of long bone

Down

2. bones made by intramembranous ossification
3. expanded end of long bone
4. ankle bones
5. joint in wrist
7. a cylinder of bone
8. _____ attaches muscle to bone
10. the early embryonic skeleton is made of this tissue
11. covers bone
12. joint which can only rotate
14. _____ attaches bone to bone
16. these bones in the thoracic cage are flat bones
17. upper arm bone

Copyright © 2020 by Pearson Education, Inc.

Name _____

CONCEPT MAP

Fill in the empty boxes with an appropriate term using the clues provided.

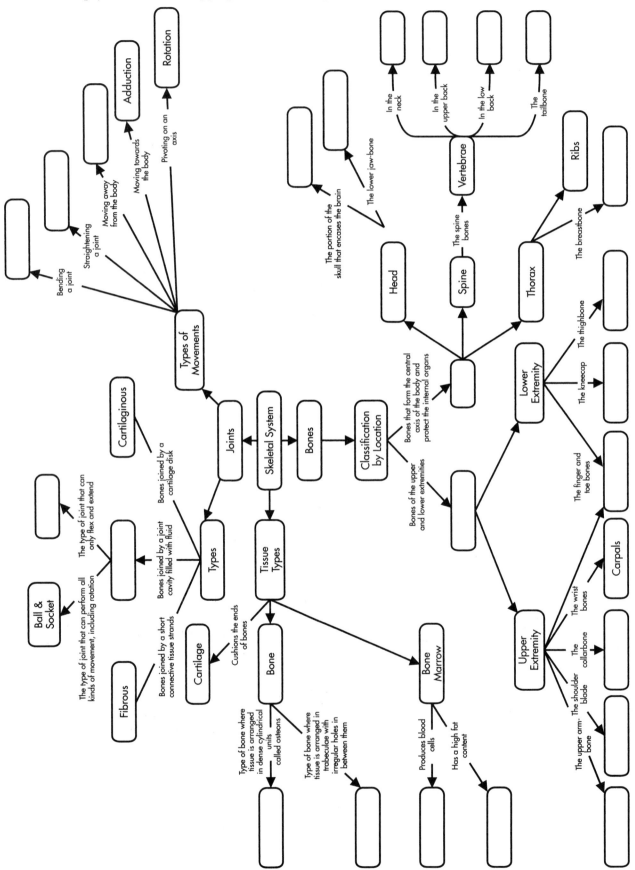

THE MUSCULAR SYSTEM: MOVEMENT FOR THE JOURNEY

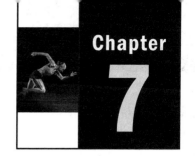

MEDICAL TERMINOLOGY REVIEW

Define the following terms.
1. Sprain: _____
2. Myalgia: _____
3. Paralysis: _____
4. Hypertrophy: _____
5. Atrophy: _____
6. Tonus: _____
7. Spasm: _____
8. Muscular dystrophy: _____
9. Electromyogram: _____
10. Strain: _____

MULTIPLE CHOICE

Circle the letter of the correct answer.
1. Choose the correct structural arrangement from macro to micro in terms of size.
   a. Muscle cell, myofibril, sarcomere, myofilament
   b. Myofibril, myofilament, muscle cell, sarcomere
   c. Myofilament, muscle cell, myofibril, sarcomere
   d. Muscle cell, myofilament, sarcomere, myofibril

2. Which of the following is a group of anterior thigh muscles?
   a. Hamstrings
   b. Quadriceps
   c. Peroneals
   d. Gluteals

3. Which of the following is a group of buttocks muscles?
   a. Psoas
   b. Gluteals
   c. Hamstrings
   d. Quadriceps

4. Which of the following is a muscle of the lower leg?
   a. Gastrocnemius
   b. Latissimus dorsi
   c. Deltoid
   d. Hamstring

5. Muscles that are used for duration or high endurance activity will:
   a. look white due to the excess oxygen and fat stored for energy
   b. look white due to the lack of blood supply
   c. look dark due to the rich blood supply to carry needed oxygen
   d. look dark due to chronic tears and scar tissue in the muscle fibers

6. Where are calcium ions stored in the muscle cells?
   a. End bulb
   b. Nucleus
   c. Myosin cross bridges
   d. Sarcoplasmic reticulum

7. Which of the following muscles are under voluntary control?
   a. Skeletal
   b. Cardiac
   c. Visceral
   d. Smooth

8. After death, when the body becomes stiff due to unreleased muscle contraction, the condition is referred to as:
   a. rigor mortis.
   b. tetanus.
   c. myalgia.
   d. paralysis.

9. When the diameter of a blood vessel increases:
   a. the pressure also increases.
   b. it is termed vasoconstriction.
   c. the pressure decreases.
   d. b and c

10. An injury or tear to a ligament is called a:
    a. strain.
    b. sprain.
    c. spasm.
    d. shin splint.

11. Which of the following is *not* a characteristic shared by the three major muscle types?
    a. Extensibility
    b. Contractility
    c. Conductivity
    d. Elasticity

12. Why are migratory bird's breasts dark (as in the King Eider, Arctic Tern, and Blue Winged Teal) and nonmigratory bird's breasts white (as in the Turkey, Sandhill Crane, and Red Cardinal)?
    a. Migratory birds need speed to traverse long distances; dark meat is a clear attribute for speed.
    b. Nonmigratory birds need endurance to traverse long distances; dark meat is a clear attribute for endurance.
    c. Migratory birds need endurance to traverse long distances; dark meat is a clear attribute for endurance.
    d. Nonmigratory birds need speed to traverse long distances; white meat is a clear attribute for endurance.

13. What is/are the energy source(s) used by muscle?
    a. Calcium
    b. Fat
    c. Glucose
    d. b and c

14. Which of the following is true about the sliding filament theory and consequently about muscle contraction?
    a. Cross-bridges are formed between actin and myosin; myosin rotates, pulling the actin toward the center of the sarcomere
    b. Cross-bridges are formed between actin and the Z-lines; Z-lines rotate, and as a result, myosin shortens
    c. Cross-bridges are formed between actin and myosin; actin rotates, pulling myosin toward the Z lines, shortening the sarcoplasmic reticulum
    d. Sarcoplasmic reticulum releases phosphorus, resulting in cross-bridges forming between myosin and the Z lines; actin rotates, pulling toward the center of the sarcomere

15. Some sphincters are examples of:
    a. skeletal muscles.
    b. smooth muscles.
    c. visceral muscle.
    d. All of the above

16. If the erector spinae muscles are the antagonist, which of the following will be a prime mover?
    a. Latissumus dorsi
    b. Trapezius
    c. Rectus abdominis
    d. a and b

17. One of the calf muscles, called the soleus, when contracted moves the heel of the foot (calcaneus) closer to the posterior leg. Given this information and your knowledge of the principles of origin and insertion, what is the muscle's origin?
    a. Calcaneus
    b. Anterior leg
    c. Posterior leg
    d. a and b

18. A group of muscles called the scalenes laterally flexes the neck. Given this information and your knowledge of the principles of origin and insertion, which of the following most likely is its insertion?
    a. Cervical vertebrae
    b. Shoulder
    c. Ribs
    d. Collarbone

19. Besides a physical separation of the thoracic cavity and the abdominal cavity, what purpose does the diaphragm serve?
    a. Flexes the trunk
    b. Extends the trunk
    c. Controls breathing
    d. All of the above

20. The diaphragm is what type of muscle?
    a. Smooth
    b. Cardiac
    c. Visceral
    d. Skeletal

21. The diaphragm is under what type of control?
    a. Voluntary
    b. Involuntary
    c. Both voluntary and involuntary
    d. Neither voluntary nor involuntary

22. A muscle called the deltoid pulls the arm away from the body, directly out away from the sides. This movement is referred to as:
    a. rotation.
    b. abduction.
    c. adduction.
    d. lateral flexion.

23. Which of the following muscles are striated?
    a. Sphincters
    b. Walls of blood vessels
    c. Muscles that move the upper arm
    d. Muscles of peristalsis

24. The gluteus maximus muscle is named for its:
    a. attachments.
    b. action.
    c. shape.
    d. size.

25. The rectus abdominis is named for its:
    a. size
    b. attachments
    c. action
    d. location

MATCHING EXERCISES

Match each term with the appropriate definition.

Set 1

_____ 1. latissimus dorsi
_____ 2. pectoralis major
_____ 3. rectus abdominis
_____ 4. erector spinae
_____ 5. orbicularis oculi
_____ 6. masseter
_____ 7. orbicularis oris
_____ 8. mentalis
_____ 9. sternocleidomastoid
_____ 10. external obliques

a. muscle encircling the mouth
b. muscle encircling the eyes
c. muscle to the side of the jaw
d. neck muscle
e. chest muscle
f. vertical muscle from inferior margin of rib cage to the pubis
g. lateral abdominal muscle
h. back muscle running from the vertebrae to the upper arm
i. vertical back muscle running from lower vertebrae to upper vertebrae
j. muscle of the midchin

Set 2

_____ 1. flexion
_____ 2. rotation
_____ 3. abduction
_____ 4. extension
_____ 5. adduction
_____ 6. vasodilate
_____ 7. vasoconstrict
_____ 8. tetanus
_____ 9. antagonist
_____ 10. agonist

a. prime mover
b. lengthens upon movement or contraction of prime mover
c. movement away from midline
d. movement toward midline
e. movement decreasing angle of the joint
f. movement increasing the angle of the joint
g. movement decreasing the diameter of the blood vessel
h. movement increasing the diameter of the blood vessels
i. movement around a center axis
j. movement that creates rigid paralysis

Set 3

_____ 1. myalgia
_____ 2. hernia
_____ 3. strain
_____ 4. cramp
_____ 5. sprain
_____ 6. myasthenia gravis
_____ 7. Guillain-Barré syndrome
_____ 8. botulism
_____ 9. atrophy
_____ 10. muscular dystrophy

a. tear or injury in muscle and/or tendon
b. involuntary, sudden, and violent contractions
c. tears or breaks in a ligament
d. a PNS disorder resulting in flaccid paralysis
e. a disorder in which patients experience progressive yet gradual muscle weakness
f. inherited muscle disease in which muscle fibers degenerate
g. a potentially deadly disease that causes paralysis and is a result of ingested bacteria
h. tenderness and pain in muscle
i. a tear in a muscle wall through which an organ protrudes
j. condition marked by rigid muscle spasm caused by a bacteria most likely entering the body via a puncture wound
k. the process of muscle wasting away; could be due to lack of nutrition, disease, or disuse

Set 4

_____ 1. triceps brachii
_____ 2. masseter
_____ 3. sternocleidomastoid
_____ 4. pectoralis major
_____ 5. deltoid
_____ 6. gluteus maximus
_____ 7. biceps brachii
_____ 8. hamstrings
_____ 9. quadriceps
_____ 10. gastrocnemius

a. flexes leg at knee
b. abducts arm
c. flexes arm at elbow
d. extends arm at elbow
e. flexes and rotates head
f. extends thigh
g. closes jaw
h. extends leg at knee
i. plantar flexes foot
j. flexes, rotates, and adducts arm

FILL IN THE BLANK

Fill in the blanks to complete the following statements.

1. Structures called _____ allow for uniform contraction of the cardiac muscle.

2. The rhythmic internal movement of food products though the GI tract is termed _____.

3. The _____ muscle is the antagonist of the biceps brachii.

4. In order to supply energy and heat, the body converts stored _____ into glucose.

5. The functional unit of the muscle is the _____.

6. Neurons secrete a neurotransmitter called _____, which sets the process of muscle contraction in motion.
7. Each functional unit of the muscle is separated from the others by _____.
8. Provided that the hamstrings are the prime movers, the _____ are the antagonists.
9. The group of muscles called the _____ assists the prime movers in a particular movement.
10. Smooth muscle is also called _____ muscle.
11. Cardiac muscle forms the walls of the _____.
12. A fibrous tissue attaching muscle to bone is a _____.
13. The deltoid muscle is named for its _____.
14. The biceps brachii is located on the _____.
15. In order for myosin heads to bind, detach, and bind again to actin, two molecules are necessary: _____ and _____.
16. The thin filaments are called _____.
17. Pain in the tibial region is a symptom of _____, a common tendon injury in runners.
18. Although easily prevented by vaccination, _____, caused by a bacteria found in the soil, can be spread by any type of skin puncture.
19. A condition in which there is lack of coordination of muscles is called _____.
20. A sprain is tearing of a _____.
21. Chronic damage to a tendon is called _____.
22. When the neurotransmitter acetylcholine binds to the receptors on the surface of skeletal muscle, _____ ions enter the muscle cell, exciting it.
23. What is stored and released from the sarcoplasmic reticulum? _____
24. Ben is hoping to beat the state record for the long jump. He runs toward the takeoff board, plants his foot, and sails into the air. Soon after takeoff, he feels a terrible pain in his extended leg. He breaks the state record, but must be carried out of the pit because his leg will not take any weight. He has torn his _____ muscle(s).
25. Wini is on the last part of the obstacle course at boot camp. She grabs the rope and swings across a stream to the platform on the other side. She lands awkwardly on the edge, injuring her ankle. Her ankle swells right away. She can gingerly put weight on the foot but an examination reveals that she cannot point her toes. She has torn her _____ tendon.

SHORT ANSWER

1. List the rules for naming skeletal muscles.

2. Explain muscle contraction.

3. How do muscles obtain energy for contraction?

4. Explain the relationship between origin, insertion, and action.

5. List and describe three types of muscle tissue.

LEARNING ACTIVITIES

1. For 10 muscles of your choice, explain how they are named based on the rules for naming muscles.

2. On a plastic or cardboard skeleton, use yarn to simulate muscle action. For the major muscles, attach one end to the insertion and pull it toward the origin. How do the origin and insertion relate to the action?

3. Play "Muscle Five Questions." One person thinks of a muscle and the other identifies the muscle described by asking up to five questions about the muscle.

4. There are many muscle-enhancing dietary supplements on the market. Using the internet, investigate one of these supplements. Is there any biological basis for the product's claims?

LABELING ACTIVITY

Label the muscles and color them for contrast. Use Figure 7–2 of your textbook as a guide.

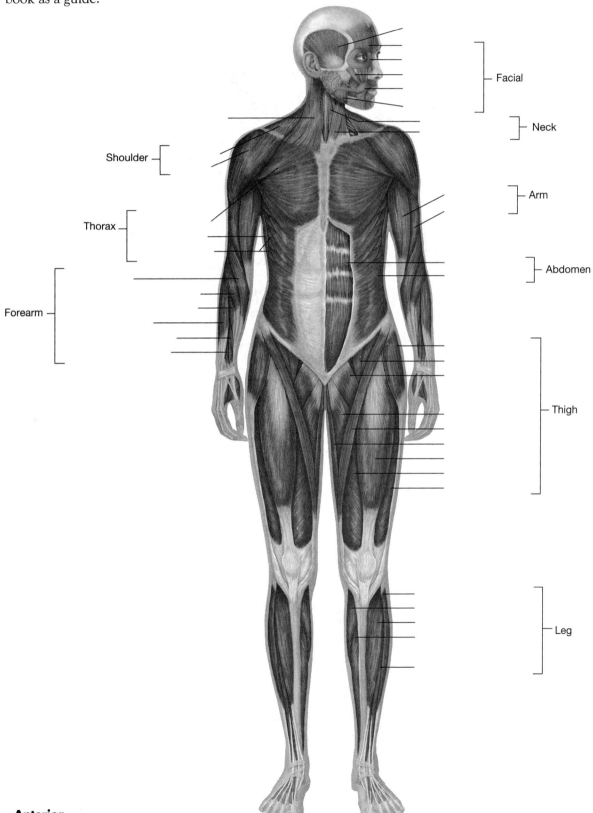

Anterior

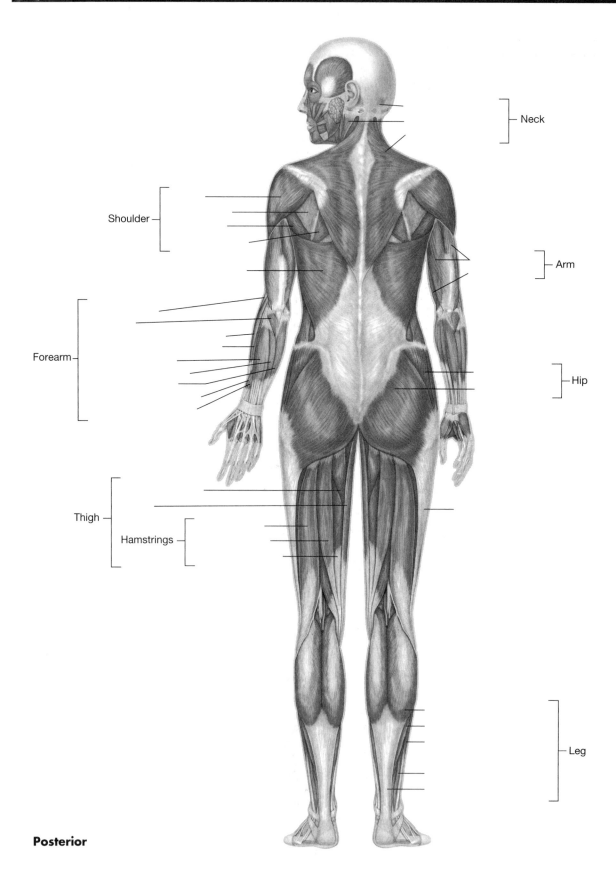

Posterior

CROSSWORD PUZZLE

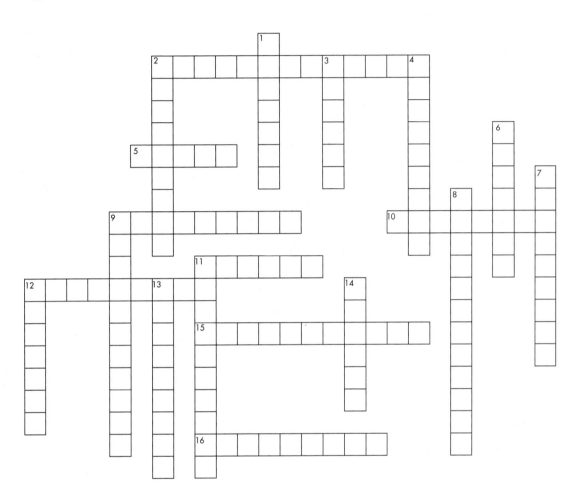

Across
2. neurotransmitter that excites skeletal muscle
5. thin filament
9. cylindrical subdivision of muscle fiber
10. spinning on axis
11. prime movement of muscle
12. movement toward center
15. sheet-like muscle attachments
16. fundamental contractile unit of muscle

Down
1. decreased joint angle
2. movement away from center
3. stationary attachments
4. increased joint angle
5. ion necessary for cross-bridge formation
6. aids primary mover
8. the _____ reticulum stores calcium
9. the medical name for a muscle cell
11. opposes the prime mover
12. prime mover
13. mobile muscle attachments
14. thick filament

Name _____

CONCEPT MAP

Fill in the empty boxes with an appropriate term using the clues provided.

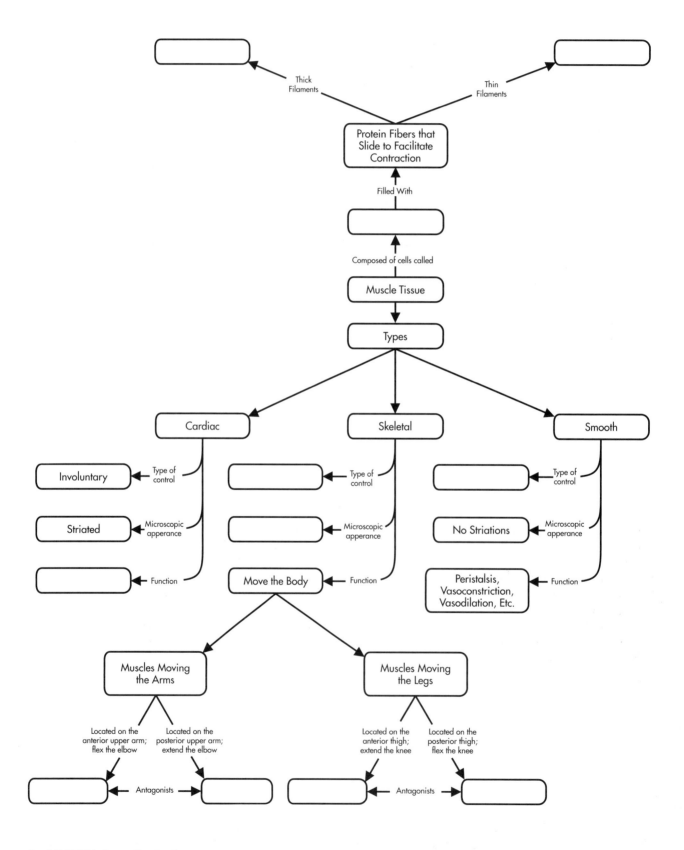

THE INTEGUMENTARY SYSTEM: THE PROTECTIVE COVERING

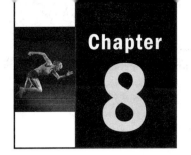

MEDICAL TERMINOLOGY REVIEW

Define the following terms.

1. Macule: _____
2. Pustule: _____
3. Wheal: _____
4. Ulcer: _____
5. Papule: _____
6. Crust: _____
7. Keloid: _____
8. Scale: _____
9. Vesicle: _____
10. Fissure: _____

MULTIPLE CHOICE

Circle the letter of the correct answer.

1. Hair is composed of a protein called:
   a. hemoglobin.
   b. lanugo.
   c. lunago.
   d. keratin.

2. The skin condition caused by the herpes simplex virus forming a visible lesion on the lip margins is called:
   a. psoriasis.
   b. pustule.
   c. cold sore.
   d. acne.

3. The cells of the epidermis are born in this layer:
   a. stratum corneum.
   b. stratum lucidum.
   c. stratum germinativum.
   d. stratum spinosum.

4. "Jock itch" is caused by which of the following?
   a. Fungi
   b. Viruses
   c. Bacteria
   d. Protozoa

5. Located in the eyelids, these glands secrete sebum into tears.
   a. Apocrine
   b. Subcutaneous
   c. Eccrine
   d. Meibomian

6. A yellowish coloration of the skin is called:
   a. keratinization.
   b. cyanosis.
   c. jaundice.
   d. freckles.

7. Acne develops when:
   a. glucose in consumed sweets solidifies in the sebaceous glands.
   b. there is an overproduction of sebum and an inflammation of the oil glands.
   c. the sweat glands are blocked with dirt and environmental grime.
   d. sweat becomes too sweet, and viruses are attracted and accumulate at the pore opening.

8. The outer layer of the epidermis contains dead cells filled with:
   a. lipids.
   b. carotene.
   c. keratin.
   d. keloids.

9. To which of the following structures do the arrector pili muscles attach?
   a. Hair follicle
   b. Stratum corneum
   c. Elastin
   d. Subcutaneous fascia

10. In order for effective body cooling to occur:
    a. water from sweat glands is excreted onto the skin, then is evaporated off, dispelling heat from the surface.
    b. water from sweat glands is excreted onto the skin, then as soon as it is felt, needs to be wiped off, carrying heat with the towel or cloth used.
    c. urination needs to cease, and excessive water consumption must be temporarily stopped.
    d. sweat needs to be at the body's core temperature, and nitrogenous wastes must be absent in the sweat excretion.

11. What determines the texture of hair?
    a. shaft shape: flat shafts produce curly hair; round shafts produce straight hair.
    b. follicle shape: vertical follicles produce straight hair; angular follicles produce curly hair.
    c. pigmentation: higher concentrations of pigmentation produce curly hair.
    d. heat and humidity: people exposed to cold will grow straight hair and people exposed to heat will not.

12. What determines the color of hair?
    a. Carotene
    b. Melanin
    c. Keratin
    d. Bilirubin

13. Shaving or frequent trimming will:
    a. cause hair to grow faster.
    b. cause hair to grow back slower.
    c. cause hair to grow back curlier.
    d. none of the above.

14. What are the three parts of hair?
    a. Cuticle, corium, and papilla
    b. Villa, erector, and lunago
    c. Shaft, body, and cuticle
    d. Follicle, root, and shaft

15. Why is vitamin D a necessity for healthy bones and teeth?
    a. It is needed for the differentiation between osteoclasts and osteoblasts.
    b. It is needed for calcium absorption in the intestine.
    c. It is needed for fighting gingivitis and calcium buildup.
    d. It is not a necessity.

16. What degree is a sunburn?
    a. First
    b. Second
    c. Third
    d. Fourth

17. Which of the following layers of skin is the deepest?
    a. Hypodermis
    b. Dermis
    c. Corium
    d. Epidermis

18. Which of the following cells pull the edges of a wound together?
    a. Red blood cells
    b. Melanocytes
    c. Fibroblasts
    d. Osteocytes

19. What role do white blood cells have in wound healing?
    a. Clotting and secreting meshlike barrier
    b. Dissolving debris by chemically breaking bond and mechanically pushing debris to the surface
    c. Fighting infection
    d. Blood thinning

20. Which of the following statements is true about melanin, melanocytes, and skin color?
    a. Adult humans, despite race or gender, have the same amount of melanocytes per skin square inch; skin color difference is due to the amount of melanin secreted from the standard number of melanocytes
    b. Different skin colors and tones are due to different amounts and arrangements of melanocytes
    c. The more melanin produced, the lighter the skin
    d. Melanocyte absolute numbers are inversely proportional to the concentration of melanin in the skin; in other words, the more melanocytes, the less pigment can be secreted and can ultimately survive in the skin

21. A clinician can estimate the extent of the area covered by a burn using what strategy?
    a. Rule of size
    b. Rule of thumb
    c. Rule of nines
    d. Color rule

22. In a condition called cirrhosis, a liver dysfunction, fair skin appears yellow, but in dark skin the yellow may not be evident. Where can the yellow color be seen?
    a. Eyes
    b. Palms
    c. Teeth
    d. Soles

23. Which of the following sweat glands secrete at the hair follicle of sebaceous glands?
    a. Sebaceous
    b. Apocrine
    c. Eccrine
    d. Creatine

24. What is the most important trigger of skin cancer?
    a. UV radiation
    b. Age
    c. Diet
    d. Lifestyle

25. What is the most important clinical concern in serious burns?
    a. Lack of pigmentation
    b. Fluid loss
    c. Hair loss
    d. Lack of sensation

MATCHING EXERCISES

Match each term with the appropriate definition.

Set 1

_____ 1. bilirubin   a. yellow jaundice
_____ 2. keratin   b. cools the body
_____ 3. fibroblasts   c. sexual attractant
_____ 4. lipocytes   d. fat
_____ 5. sebum   e. oil
_____ 6. carotene   f. true skin
_____ 7. melanin   g. found in hair and nails
_____ 8. corium   h. skin healing
_____ 9. apocrine   i. darkening of the skin
_____ 10. eccrine   j. natural yellow hue to the skin

Set 2

_____ 1. cuticle   a. hypodermis
_____ 2. dermis   b. encloses hair root
_____ 3. sebaceous   c. layer in which epidermal cells are born
_____ 4. lunula   d. lubricates and moisturizes hair and skin
_____ 5. sudoriferous   e. adheres nail body to nail bed
_____ 6. stratum basale   f. contractile tissue associated with hair follicle
_____ 7. subcutaneous   g. covers nail root
_____ 8. matrix   h. contains glands, vessels, collagen, and elastic fibers
_____ 9. hair follicle   i. excretes water and nitrogenous wastes
_____ 10. arrector pili   j. proximal, whitish, half-moon part of nail

Set 3

_____ 1. freckles   a. herpes zoster
_____ 2. acne   b. patches of excessive melanin production
_____ 3. urticaria   c. herpes simplex
_____ 4. psoriasis   d. cancer
_____ 5. fever blister   e. hives
_____ 6. shingles   f. open necrotic sore
_____ 7. eczema   g. itching, scaling, redness, circular borders
_____ 8. abrasion   h. superficial form of dermatitis
_____ 9. ulcer   i. rubbing off or scratching off of the skin
_____ 10. malignant melanoma j. infection of the sebaceous gland

Set 4

_____ 1. dermatitis
_____ 2. scabies
_____ 3. urticaria
_____ 4. contusion
_____ 5. athlete's foot
_____ 6. burn
_____ 7. decubitus ulcer
_____ 8. abrasion
_____ 9. pustule
_____ 10. malignant melanoma

a. fungal infection
b. touching poison ivy
c. heat, radiation, chemicals
d. UV radiation
e. egg-laying mites
f. infected hair follicle
g. extended pressure on skin
h. allergic reaction
i. mechanical scraping of skin
j. mechanical damage to skin

FILL IN THE BLANK

Fill in the blanks to complete the following statements.

1. Located in the middle layer of the skin, _____ fibers help the skin flex with the movement of the body.
2. The most dangerous and life threatening of the skin cancers is _____.
3. Shingles, caused by the _____ virus, are found mainly on the torso or trunk of the body.
4. The skin muscles that contract, indirectly forming what is commonly known as gooseflesh or goose bumps, are called _____.
5. The _____ layer of the epidermis is constantly shedding as a part of the skin replacement process.
6. The clinical term for pimple is _____.
7. A human adult, having thousands of sweat glands per square inch, has the potential of excreting up to _____ liters of sweat in 24 hours.
8. Normally, it takes _____ seconds to re-perfuse the nail bed when assessing perfusion of the extremity by squeezing the nail.
9. When a person has an injury that does not break the skin yet damages the underlying small blood vessels, this person has experienced a(n) _____.
10. "Dry skin" refers to the lack of _____.
11. The most severe of the burns, _____ degree burn, is marked by tissue damage from the skin's surface to the bone.
12. The patient has experienced _____ percent body-surface-area damage when both upper and lower limbs, the neck, and the head are burned.
13. Nails grow from the nail _____.
14. The substance or pigment responsible for the darkening of the skin is _____.

15. In hepatitis, a liver disease, _____ builds up in the blood, giving the skin an unhealthy yellowish color.
16. A(n) _____ is a pathologically altered patch of skin.
17. _____ is a genetic pigment disorder in which a person's body cells do not produce the usual amounts of melanin.
18. The reawakening of dormant chicken pox years later is known as _____.
19. A third degree burn penetrates through the _____.
20. The upper 20 percent of the _____ is called the papillary layer and is attached to the epidermis.
21. Anything that is under the skin is called _____.
22. Two characteristics are used to evaluate burns: the _____ of the burn and the _____ of skin involved.
23. Bob catches strep throat from his niece. His doctor gives him a new antibiotic for the infection. A few days into the medication, he develops a red, raised itchy rash. This kind of a skin reaction to medication is called _____.
24. Alice is confined to bed after a car accident. She develops an infected _____ ulcer.
25. One function of skin is _____.

SHORT ANSWER

1. Explain the journey of epidermal cells from birth to death.
   _____
   _____
   _____
   _____

2. Contrast the three types of skin cancer in terms of severity and depth.
   _____
   _____
   _____
   _____

3. How do pressure ulcers (bedsores) develop?
   _____
   _____
   _____
   _____

4. Besides vitamin D production, what are three functions of skin?

   _____

   _____

   _____

   _____

5. Explain the classification of burns.

   _____

   _____

   _____

   _____

LEARNING ACTIVITIES

1. The textbook could not possibly cover all skin diseases. Use the Internet to research some diseases of the skin you haven't read about. What else can go wrong with skin?
2. Many older adults go to great lengths to fight the effects of aging on skin, having face-lifts and dermabrasion treatment, getting Botox injections, coloring their hair to hide gray, or replacing lost hair. Use the Internet to research what happens to skin and hair as people age.
3. Write a scenario in which a patient is burned, describing the depth and extent of the burn. Use the rule of nines and the degree system to diagnose the severity of the burn.
4. There are many accessory structures in the skin. List them and their contribution to skin function. Can you list them all?

LABELING ACTIVITY

Label and color code the various structures of the skin. Use Figure 8–1 of your textbook as a guide.

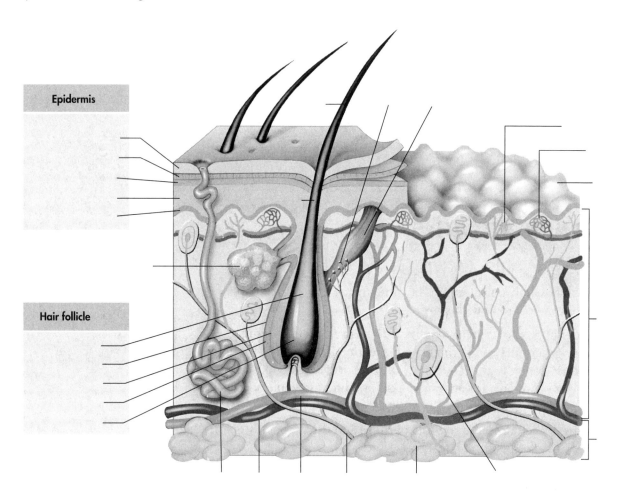

Epidermis

Hair follicle

CROSSWORD PUZZLE

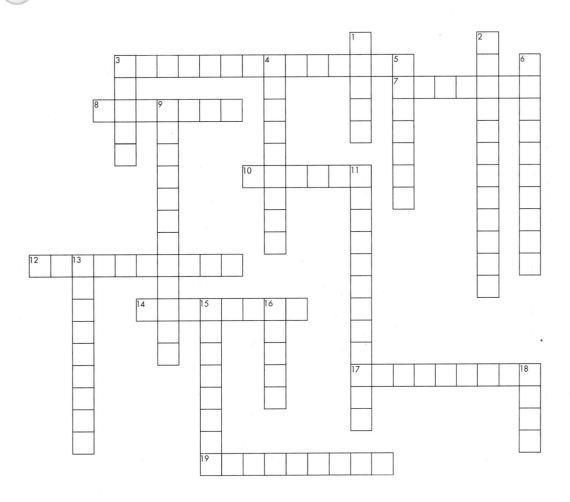

Across

3. the outer layer of dead epidermal cells
7. sweat glands which help regulate body temperature
8. hardened protein found in hair and nails
10. layer of skin with connective tissue and accessory structures
12. deepest skin layer
14. made when skin is exposed to sunlight (2 words)
17. _____ glands secrete oil
19. surface layer of skin

Down

1. Burns can be categorized by _____ and extent
2. hair grows from cells in the _____ (2 words)
3. secreted when body temperature rises
4. pertaining to skin
5. dark skin pigment
6. melanoma is cancer of this cell
9. contraction of this muscle makes hair stand on end (2 words)
11. epidermal cells are born here
13. _____ is monitored using the nails
15. secretes a sexual attractant
16. extent of burn injury is determined using rule of _____
18. medical term is integument

Name _____

CONCEPT MAP

Fill in the empty boxes with an appropriate term using the clues provided.

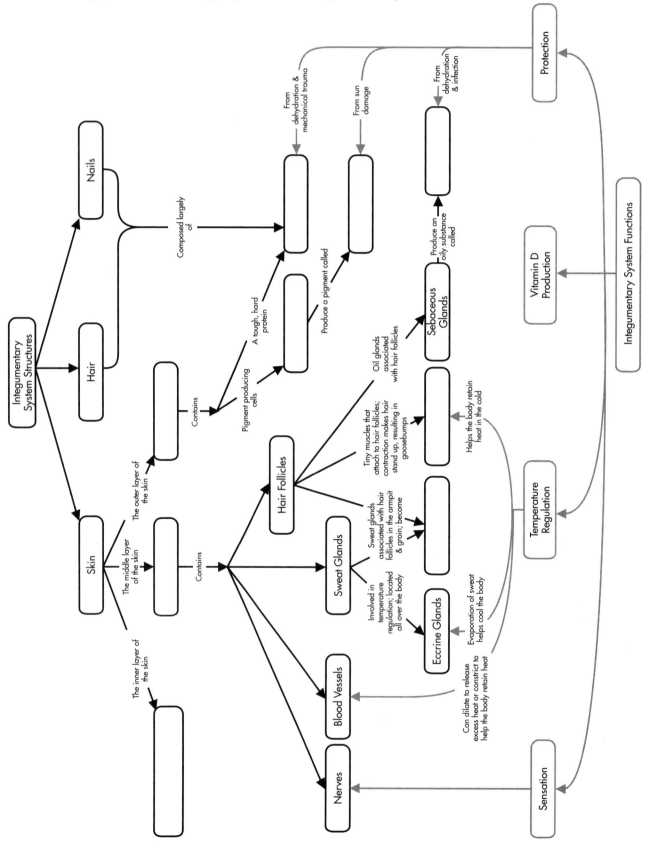

THE NERVOUS SYSTEM (PART I): THE INFORMATION SUPER HIGHWAY

MEDICAL TERMINOLOGY REVIEW

Define the following terms.
1. Neuropathy: _____
2. Paralysis: _____
3. Spinal cord injury: _____
4. Carpal tunnel syndrome: _____
5. Multiple sclerosis: _____
6. Guillain-Barré syndrome: _____
7. Meningitis: _____
8. Myasthenia gravis: _____
9. Paraplegia: _____
10. Quadriplegia: _____

MULTIPLE CHOICE

Circle the letter of the correct answer.

1. The function of the lateral horn is:
   a. fusing the spinal nerves.
   b. autonomic control.
   c. communication between multipolar motor neurons and bipolor motor neurons.
   d. serving as a superhighway for myelinated neurons up and down the spinal cord.

2. What is the name for the lumbar, sacral, and coccygeal spinal nerves that dangle in the vertebral canal from the bottom of the spinal cord?
   a. Equinal ropa
   b. Cauda equina
   c. Equine threades
   d. Linea alba

3. What two structures make up the entire central nervous system?
   a. Spinal cord and spinal nerve
   b. Gray and white matter
   c. Brain and spinal cord
   d. Brachial and lumbar plexuses

4. What do both sets of spinal roots fuse to form?
   a. Spinal cord
   b. Spinal nerve
   c. Ganglion
   d. Conus medullaris

5. The chemical that inhibits the release of pain neurotransmitter is:
   a. calcium.
   b. serotonin.
   c. sarin.
   d. endorphin.

6. Where does the spinal cord end?
   a. Lumbar 2 vertebra
   b. Coccygeal 3 vertebra
   c. Plexus 5 vertebra
   d. Medulla oblongata

7. The dorsal horn of the spinal cord is involved with:
   a. production of cerebral spinal fluid.
   b. motor function.
   c. sensory function.
   d. coordination.

8. Choose the correct order of the CNS's protective membrane from innermost to outermost layer.
   a. Pia mater, dura mater, arachnoid
   b. Archnoid, dura mater, pia mater
   c. Pia mater, arachnoid, dura mater
   d. Dura mater, arachnoid, pia mater

9. Severe damage to the spinal cord at the lumbar level may result in:
   a. quadriplegia.
   b. blindness.
   c. bipedalism.
   d. paraplegia.

10. How many nerves enter and exit at the cervical region?
    a. 31
    b. 6
    c. 24
    d. 8

11. In the CNS, the glial cells that cover surfaces and line cavities are called:
    a. ependymal cells.
    b. oligodendrocytes.
    c. Schwann cells.
    d. astrocytes.

12. How many pairs of spinal nerves does the average child have between 13 and 18 years of age?
    a. 31
    b. 29
    c. 17
    d. 24

13. The combination of axon terminal and receiving muscle cell is called:
    a. node of Ranvier.
    b. dendrite.
    c. neuromuscular junction.
    d. cordae tendinae.

14. Which of the following is the part of the neuron that functions in cell metabolism?
    a. Axon terminal
    b. Cell body
    c. Vesicle
    d. Sympathetic

15. The nervous system has an output side called:
    a. motor.
    b. sensory.
    c. association.
    d. neuroglia.

16. Besides the size of the axon, what other characteristic is a determinant of impulse speed down the axon?
    a. The concentration of the neurotransmitter
    b. Dendritic branches
    c. Myelination
    d. Lack of dendritic branches

17. For repolarization to occur, which of the following is true about movement of ions?
    a. Potassium moves out of cells
    b. Calcium moves into cell
    c. Sodium moves into cell
    d. Chlorine moves out of cell

18. Which of the following neurotransmitters can be found in the CNS, PNS, and mainly at skeletal neuromuscular synapses?
    a. Norepinephrine
    b. Acetylcholine
    c. Epinephrine
    d. Serotonin

19. Between Schwann cells are bare spots where channels must open in order for an action potential to flow rapidly down the axon. What are they called?
    a. Nodes of Ranvier
    b. Conus medullaris
    c. Myelin
    d. Spudus impulsasis

20. When the axon terminal depolarizes, what kind of ions flow in, causing exocytosis?
    a. Sodium
    b. Calcium
    c. Acetylcholine
    d. Potassium
21. Which one of the following systems controls smooth muscle, cardiac muscle, and glands?
    a. Somatic nervous system
    b. Sensory system
    c. Autonomic nervous system
    d. All of the above
22. Which of the following branches in the body's alert system is commonly known as "fight or flight"?
    a. Sympathetic
    b. Parasympathetic
    c. Central nervous system
    d. a and b
23. The part of the neuron that functions to receive information from other cells or the environment is called:
    a. axon.
    b. vesicle.
    c. dendrite.
    d. Schwann.
24. Multipolar neurons can be described as:
    a. many cell bodies; single dendrite, single axon.
    b. unlimited ionic transferability.
    c. many dendrites, single axon.
    d. one dendrite, multiple axons.
25. With a neuron at rest, which of the following is true about the charges inside and outside the cell?
    a. Inside the cell has a positive charge, whereas outside the cell has a negative charge
    b. Both inside and outside the cell have positive charges
    c. Inside the cell has a negative charge, whereas outside the cell has a positive charge
    d. Both inside and outside the cell have negative charges

MATCHING EXERCISES

Match each term with the appropriate definition.

Set 1

_____ 1. meningitis
_____ 2. polarized
_____ 3. botulism
_____ 4. Guillian-Barré syndrome
_____ 5. paralyzed diaphragm
_____ 6. multiple sclerosis
_____ 7. diabetes and alcoholism
_____ 8. myasthenia gravis
_____ 9. polio and shingles
_____ 10. carpal tunnel syndrome

a. paralysis of four chambers of the heart
b. systemic, may cause peripheral neuropathy
c. inflammation of the peripheral nerves leading to rapid onset of paralysis (no known cause)
d. caused by ingested bacteria, resulting in paralysis
e. autoimmune disorder in which acetylcholine receptors are reduced
f. lead(s) to respiratory arrest
g. flexor tendon sheath becomes inflamed compressing a wrist nerve
h. infections that may cause peripheral neuropathy
i. viral or bacterial infection of the lining of the brain and spinal cord
j. not stimulated; not excited
k. damage to the myelin sheath, leading to poor impulse conductivity

Set 2

1. neuron
2. astrocytes
3. satellite cells
4. dura mater
5. microglia
6. arachnoid mater
7. Schwann
8. oligodendrocyte
9. pia mater
10. ependymal cells

a. precursor of neuroglial cells
b. metabolic and structural support cells of the CNS
c. support(s) cells of PNS
d. nerve cells for functional control of the nervous system
e. cover(s) surfaces and lines cavities of the CNS
f. innermost meningeal layer
g. outermost meningeal layer
h. middle meningeal layer
i. cells that remove debris from the CNS
j. make(s) myelin for the CNS
k. make(s) myelin for the PNS

Set 3

1. endorphin
2. acetylcholine
3. serotonin
4. norepinephrine
5. tetrodotoxin
6. calcium
7. potassium
8. sarin
9. acetylcholinesterase
10. sodium

a. inhibits acetylcholinesterase; used by terrorist on Tokyo's subways
b. breaks downs ACh
c. triggers the release of neurotransmitters from the vesicles
d. inhibits the release of pain neurotransmitters
e. skeletal neuromuscular junction neurotransmitter
f. poison in fugu
g. regulates temperature, mood, and onset of sleep
h. increases heart rate and blood pressure
i. rushes out of cells for repolarization to occur
j. rushes into the cell for depolarization

Set 4

1. dorsal root ganglion
2. ventral horn
3. commissure
4. ascending tracts
5. descending tracts
6. lateral horn
7. spinal nerves
8. gray matter
9. white matter
10. central canal

a. motor neurons
b. carry(ies) motor information
c. autonomic neurons
d. fluid-filled center of spinal cord
e. sensory neurons
f. cell bodies
g. connect(s) right and left halves
h. carry(ies) mixed information
i. axons
j. carry(ies) sensory information

FILL IN THE BLANK

Fill in the blanks to complete the following statements.

1. The parasympathetic division of the nervous system is often called the _____ and _____ system.
2. The combination of axon terminal and receiving neural dendrite is called _____.
3. The vesicles at the axon terminal are filled with chemicals called _____.
4. The three horns of the spinal cord are the _____, the _____, and the _____ horns.
5. During labor, a woman may ask for an injection of local anesthesia called a(n) _____, which is administered between the vertebrae and the _____.
6. The spinal cord is divided in half by a(n) _____ and a(n) _____.
7. A pointed structure called the _____ marks the end of the spinal cord.
8. The _____ root is sensory, whereas the _____ root is motor.
9. The simplest form of motor output that protects us from harm is a(n) _____.
10. In carpal tunnel syndrome, the _____ nerve is affected due to swelling at the wrist.
11. Neurotransmitter is released from neurons via _____.
12. The three protective membranes of both the spinal cord and brain are called the _____.
13. A nerve cell is said to be _____ when it is stimulated.
14. When a nerve cell is stimulated, _____ ions rush into the cell.
15. A disorder called _____ is marked by myelin destruction in various areas of the CNS.
16. The _____ nerve projects from the cervical plexus and carries impulses to the diaphragm.
17. Ascending spinal cord tracts carry _____ information.
18. Fine touch information is carried by the _____ tract.
19. The corticospinal tract carries information from the brain to the _____ of the spinal cord.

20. Ari is injured in a parachute accident. He is left without sensation or movement below his armpits. His injury is in the _____ section of the spinal cord.

21. Cerebrospinal fluid (CSF) acts as a(n) _____ _____ for both the brain and the spinal cord.

22. If a spinal cord injury occurs above _____, the patient will often be ventilator dependent.

23. A neuron that is more negative than at rest is said to be _____.

24. White matter indicates the presence of _____.

25. The CSF-filled space in the spinal cord is the _____.

SHORT ANSWER

1. Explain why myelin increases impulse conduction speed.

2. Explain the events in an action potential.

3. Explain the steps in chemical synaptic transmission.

4. List and explain the parts of a reflex.

5. What is the primary difference between action potential and graded potential?

   _____

   _____

   _____

   _____

LEARNING ACTIVITIES

1. Stem cells have been promoted as a potential cure for degenerative diseases. Choose one progressive neurological disease and research the role of stem cells as a potential treatment. How close are scientists to using stem cells to treat these disorders? Have each student in your group select a different disease and explain the role of stem cells in treatment.

2. Play "Neuro Concentration." Make a deck of cards. On one card print a nervous system structure. On the matching card print the function. Turn the cards over, keeping the ones that match.

LABELING ACTIVITY

Label the parts of the nervous system. Use Figure 5–10 from your textbook as a guide.

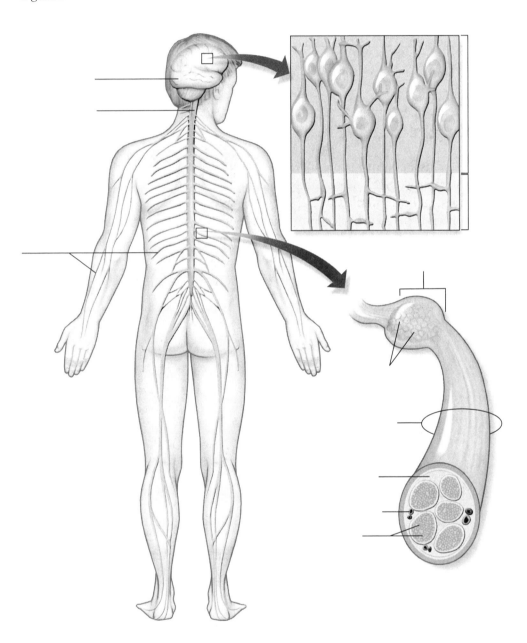

CROSSWORD PUZZLE

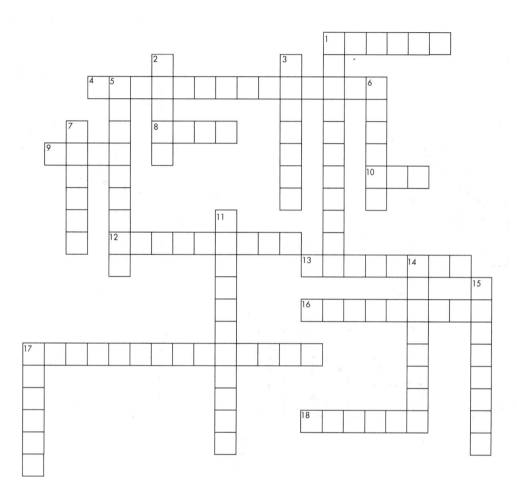

Across

1. this ion is important during depolarization
4. cell returns to resting
8. during repolarization, potassium channels _____
9. motor neurons in the spinal cord are in the ventral _____
10. during hyperpolarization, potassium moves _____ of the cell
12. general support cell for CNS
13. dura mater, arachnoid mater, and pia mater
16. action potentials do not change size, they are _____ (3 words)
17. change in cell charge that is proportional to stimulus (2 words)
18. made by oligodendrocytes

Down

1. this is formed by the fusion of dorsal and ventral roots (2 words)
2. nervous system output
3. enters the axon terminal during depolarization
5. _____ cells line CNS cavities
6. cell which sends, receives, and processes information
7. runs up and down the spinal cord
11. makes myelin for PNS (2 words)
14. collection of neurons outside CNS
15. the phrenic nerve projects from the _____ spinal cord
17. lower back

Name _____

CONCEPT MAP

Fill in the empty boxes with an appropriate term using the clues provided.

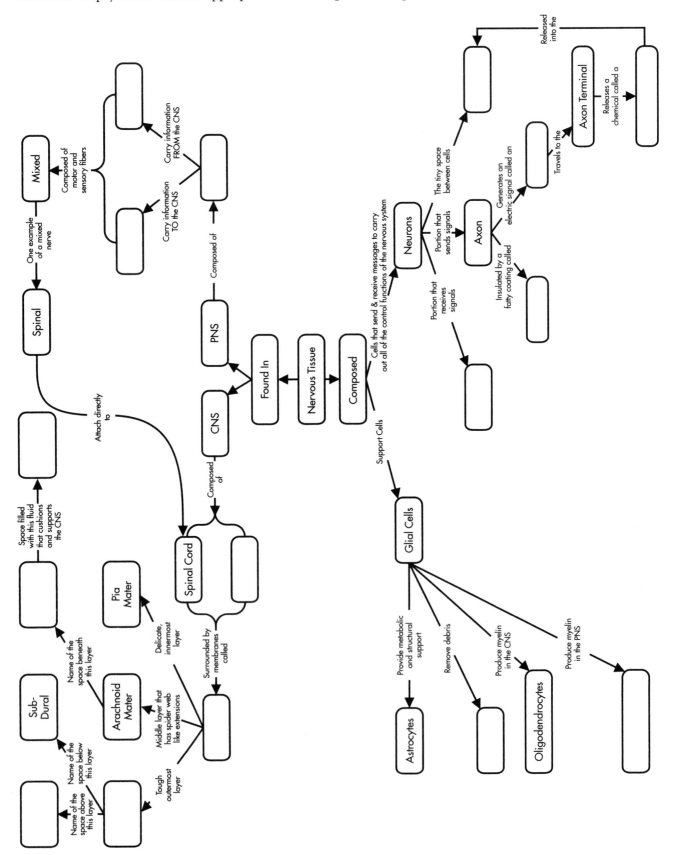

THE NERVOUS SYSTEM (PART II): THE TRAFFIC CONTROL CENTER

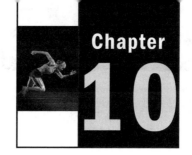

MEDICAL TERMINOLOGY REVIEW

Define the following terms.
1. Spastic: _____
2. Flaccid: _____
3. Cerebral palsy: _____
4. Cerebral vascular accident: _____
5. Coma: _____
6. Traumatic brain injury: _____
7. Huntington's disease: _____
8. Parkinson's disease: _____
9. Hydrocephalus: _____
10. Concussion: _____

MULTIPLE CHOICE

Circle the letter of the correct answer.

1. The area of the cerebral cortex that allows understanding and interpretation of somatic sensory information is called:
   a. somatic sensory association area.
   b. precentral gyrus.
   c. diencephalon.
   d. limbic reticular formation.

2. The map size in the motor cortex is proportional to the:
   a. amount of movement control.
   b. size of the structure.
   c. blood supply.
   d. insula.

3. The limbic system is located:
   a. along craniosacral divisions of the spinal cord.
   b. in the cerebellum.
   c. in the cerebrum.
   d. in the medulla.

4. If you violently stub your toe (pain), which of the following pathways carries the information to the brain?
   a. Dorsal column tract
   b. Spinothalamic tract
   c. Spinocerebellar tract
   d. Spinobulbar tract

5. Which of the following cranial nerves innervates the skeletal muscles that move the eyeballs?
   a. Trochlear
   b. Abducens
   c. Optic
   d. a and b

6. Where is the arbor vitae located?
   a. The pons
   b. The cerebrum
   c. The midbrain
   d. The cerebellum

7. How many pairs of cranial nerves do humans have?
   a. 5
   b. 7
   c. 12
   d. 31

8. The diencephalon is made up of which of the following structures?
   a. Pineal body, hypothalamus, pituitary gland, and thalamus
   b. Pineal body, cerebellum, pituitary gland, and corpus callosum
   c. Midbrain, thalamus, hypothalamus, and cerebellum
   d. Pineal body, pituitary gland, adrenal gland, and midbrain

9. What do the parasympathetic postganglionic neurons and the sympathetic preganglionic neurons secrete?
   a. Norepinephrine/epinephrine
   b. Acetylcholine/acetylcholine
   c. Epinephrine/acetylcholine
   d. Acetylcholine/norepinephrine

10. The temporal lobes are mainly responsible for:
    a. motor activities.
    b. hearing.
    c. vision.
    d. integration of emotions.

11. How many frontal lobes do humans have?
    a. 1
    b. 2
    c. 2 pairs
    d. 4 pairs

12. Where is cerebral spinal fluid made?
    a. In the arachnoid and subdural and central canals by the pituitary glands
    b. In the fourth ventricle by the cerebral aqueduct
    c. In the lateral ventricle(s) by the choroid plexus
    d. In the hypothalamus by the thalamal peptides

13. What separates the frontal lobe from the rest of the brain?
    a. The insula
    b. Central sulcus
    c. Lateral fissure
    d. Latitudinal fissure

14. The motor area for speech is:
    a. Wernicke's area.
    b. Laurel's area.
    c. Insula's area.
    d. Broca's area.

15. The function of the cerebellum is:
    a. reflex center for cough and sneeze.
    b. motor coordination and balance.
    c. coordination of heart rate with breathing rate.
    d. interpretation of crude touch and temperature.

16. Where is the cerebellum?
    a. Inferior to the medulla
    b. Posterior to the brain stem
    c. Between the thalamus and hypothalamus
    d. Superior to the midbrain

17. The function of the midbrain is:
    a. coordination.
    b. two-way conduction system pathway to relay visual and auditory impulses.
    c. wisdom, moderation of impulse, and conscience.
    d. production of cerebral spinal fluid.

18. Where is the pineal body located?
    a. Posterior to the thalamus between the corpus callosum and cerebellum
    b. Inferior to the cerebellum between the medulla and the pons
    c. Between the cerebrum and the corpus callosum
    d. Anterior and inferior to the hypothalamus

19. Ventricles of the brain are:
    a. networks of association neurons that link all four named lobes to each other.
    b. hollows or spaces in the brain for sound resonance and to make the brain lighter.
    c. ridges and crevices on the surface of the brain.
    d. fluid-filled cavities.

20. Where is the third ventricle?
    a. Between the cerebrum and the brain stem
    b. In the cerebrum between the frontal and parietal lobes
    c. In the cerebrum spanning the temporal, frontal, and parietal lobes
    d. Between the cerebellum and the medulla

21. What may cause CSF to accumulate in the brain?
    a. Blockage of passages between the cavities in the brain
    b. Tumors
    c. Decreased reabsorption
    d. All of the above

22. What effect does acetylcholine have on visceral muscles?
    a. No effect
    b. Inhibits
    c. Excites
    d. Harms

23. The smell of citrus causes Mary to feel anxious. When Mary was a child, her grandmother, who was verbally abusive, served fresh orange juice in the morning before her predictable morning tantrum. What system of the brain coordinates emotion and sense of smell as well as retrieves memories?
    a. Limbic
    b. Sympathetic
    c. Parasympathetic
    d. Somatic sensory

24. Where are the parasympathetic ganglia located?
    a. In the thoracic and lumbar segments of the spinal cord
    b. In the brain stem and sacral segments of the spinal cord
    c. Close to the visceral or glandular organs they affect
    d. Running parallel to the vertebral column/spinal cord

25. Where are the sympathetic preganglionic neurons located?
    a. In the thoracic and lumbar segments of the spinal cord
    b. In the cranial and sacral segments of the spinal cord
    c. Close to the organs or glands they affect
    d. Running parallel to the vertebral column/spinal cord

MATCHING EXERCISES

Match each term with the appropriate definition.

Set 1

_____ 1. traumatic brain injury
_____ 2. parasympathetic
_____ 3. meningitis
_____ 4. hydrocephalus
_____ 5. cerebral vascular accident
_____ 6. sympathetic
_____ 7. flaccid paralysis
_____ 8. Huntington's disease
_____ 9. cerebral palsy
_____ 10. spastic paralysis

a. thoracolumbar
b. hypertonia
c. nonprogressive childhood disease marked by motor deficits
d. hypotonia
e. damage that occurs when force is applied to the skull
f. dysfunction in which nonsterile water seeps into the brain
g. blood accumulation superficial to the arachnoid
h. inflammation of the brain and spinal cord covering
i. hereditary disorder marked by loss of cognitive function
j. stroke
k. craniosacral
l. increased accumulation of CSF in the ventricles

Set 2

_____ 1. medulla oblongata
_____ 2. parietal lobes
_____ 3. hypothalamus
_____ 4. pineal body
_____ 5. frontal lobe
_____ 6. cerebellum
_____ 7. corpus callosum
_____ 8. temporal lobe
_____ 9. pons
_____ 10. occipital lobes

a. secretes epinephrine
b. connects left and right hemispheres
c. primary area for hearing function
d. primary area for motor function
e. divides the brain into hemispheres
f. primary area for vision functions
g. coordination
h. relays sensory and motor information
i. regulates heart rate, blood pressure, vomiting
j. regulates body temperature, fear, and pleasure
k. secretes melatonin
l. primary area for sensory functions

Set 3

____ 1. facial nerve
____ 2. oculomotor nerve
____ 3. glossopharyngeal nerve
____ 4. accessory nerve
____ 5. olfactory nerve
____ 6. trochlear nerve
____ 7. optic nerve
____ 8. hypoglossal nerve
____ 9. trigeminal nerve
____ 10. vagus nerve

a. vision
b. movement of the eye, CN IV
c. sensation of the face and muscles for chewing
d. muscles of expression like squinting and smiling
e. smell
f. swallowing and taste, CN IX
g. movement of the tongue
h. movement of the shoulder's trapezius muscles
i. movement of the eye, CN III
j. sensation of the stomach (belly ache)
k. hearing and balance

Set 4

____ 1. Wernicke's area
____ 2. Broca's area
____ 3. precentral gyrus
____ 4. postcentral gyrus
____ 5. basal nuclei
____ 6. limbic system
____ 7. thalamus
____ 8. insula
____ 9. premotor cortex
____ 10. somatic sensory association area

a. motor coordination nuclei
b. relay center for motor and sensory information
c. autonomic nervous system
d. motor area for speech
e. interpreting touch information
f. understanding language, sensory interpretation
g. motor planning
h. nuclei that control emotion, mood, memory
i. primary somatic sensory cortex
j. primary motor cortex

FILL IN THE BLANK

Fill in the blanks to complete the following statements.

1. From the outside, you can see that the brain consists of three parts: the _____, _____, and _____.

2. The right and left hemispheres of the brain are divided by the _____ fissure.

3. The surface of the cerebrum has broken ridges called _____.

4. The two cranial nerves involved in taste are the _____ and the _____ nerves.

5. The occipital lobes are responsible for _____.

6. The dividing line called the _____ separates the temporal lobe from the rest of the brain.

7. The _____ contains visual and auditory reflex centers.

8. The layer of gray matter surrounding the white matter of the brain is called the _____.
9. The insula is located deep within the _____ of the brain.
10. The ventricles of the brain contain _____.
11. Position and postural sensory information are carried in the _____ pathway of the somatic sensory system.
12. The sympathetic division of the autonomic nervous system stimulates the _____ gland to secrete epinephrine.
13. A remarkable woman named Harriet Tubman was born into slavery but had the courage to free herself, hundreds of kidnapped Africans, and their descendants. Ironically, considering that she was constantly and dangerously on the run, she suffered from narcolepsy, which means she would fall asleep uncontrollably. As a child, due to a violent blow by the plantation overseer, Harriet Tubman's _____ _____ in the brain stem was damaged. This part of the brain is vital in the maintenance of conscious awareness.
14. Of the two divisions of the autonomic nervous system, the _____ controls homeostasis.
15. The corticospinal and corticobulbar tracts carry _____ signals to synaptic junctions in the ventral horn of the spinal cord.
16. Blockage or narrowing of passages between ventricles leads to a condition known as _____, which literally means "water in the head."
17. _____ are a series of minor strokes that cause temporary symptoms.
18. _____ is a genetic disease causing movement problems and dementia.
19. Mabel, a 75-year-old woman awakens one morning unable to speak or move her right side. She has had a major stroke affecting the _____ side of her cerebral cortex.
20. After a blow to the back of the head, Joe experiences dizziness and decreased coordination. What part of his brain might be damaged? _____
21. Deep islands of gray matter are called _____.
22. A(n) _____ is a collection of neurons outside the CNS.
23. Most of the cranial nerves are attached to this part of the brain _____.
24. Areas of the brain that attach meaning to sensory information are called _____ areas.
25. The _____ space contains CSF.

SHORT ANSWER

1. What is meant by *contralateral* information entering and leaving the brain?

2. Explain the role of subcortical structures in the motor system.

3. What is the purpose of brain convolutions?

4. Besides location, what are two differences between the spinal nerves and the cranial nerves?

5. What effects do the sympathetic and parasympathetic nervous systems have on skeletal muscle, cardiac muscle, and the muscle surrounding the digestive tract?

LEARNING ACTIVITIES

1. For each brain region list the deficits that would result after CVA.

2. Stem cells have been promoted as a potential cure for degenerative diseases. Choose one progressive neurological disease and research the role of stem cells as a potential treatment. How close are scientists to using stem cells to treat these disorders? Each student in the group should select a different disease and explain the role of stem cells in treatment.

3. Many well known individuals, especially athletes, have experienced neurological disorders or injuries. Do some research using the internet or news sources. What happens to a person after diagnosis of a neurological disorder, even if he or she has the best treatment? How does he cope? What happens to her? Some examples: Robin Williams, Christopher Reeve, Muhammad Ali, Lou Gehrig, Andre Waters, Ronald Reagan, and Michael J. Fox.

4. In 1982, several heroin addicts in California were poisoned by a chemical called MPTP and got instant, profound Parkinson's. Read their story. How did they develop Parkinson's? How did their illness increase our understanding of Parkinson's? (Hint: Search for "frozen addicts.")

LABELING ACTIVITY

Label and color code these three illustrations. Use your textbook as a guide.

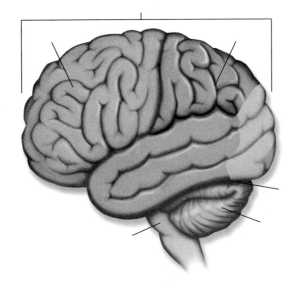

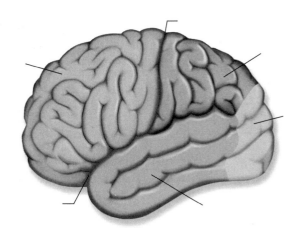

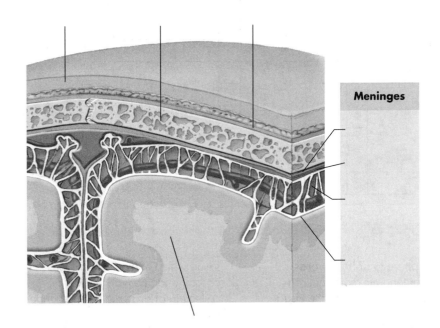

Meninges

CROSSWORD PUZZLE

Across

4. connects left hemisphere to right (2 words)
8. this horn contains autonomic motor neurons
9. the occipital _____ contains the visual cortex
12. planning is accomplished in this lobe
14. areas which add meaning to sensation
15. map in the postcentral gyrus is determined by _____ of body
17. largest part of brain
19. location of parasympathetic preganglionic neurons

Down

1. tissue which makes cerebrospinal fluid (2 words)
2. coordination network (2 words)
3. collection of gray matter surrounded by white
4. outer layer of gray matter
5. a motor homunculus is found in the _____ gyrus
6. frontal and parietal lobes are separated by the central _____
7. the _____ system controls emotion, mood and memory
10. medulla oblongata, pons, midbrain
11. abbreviation for fluid found in ventricles
13. cranial nerve II
16. cranial nerve which controls viscera
18. motor area for speech

Name _____

CONCEPT MAP

Fill in the empty boxes with an appropriate term using the clues provided.

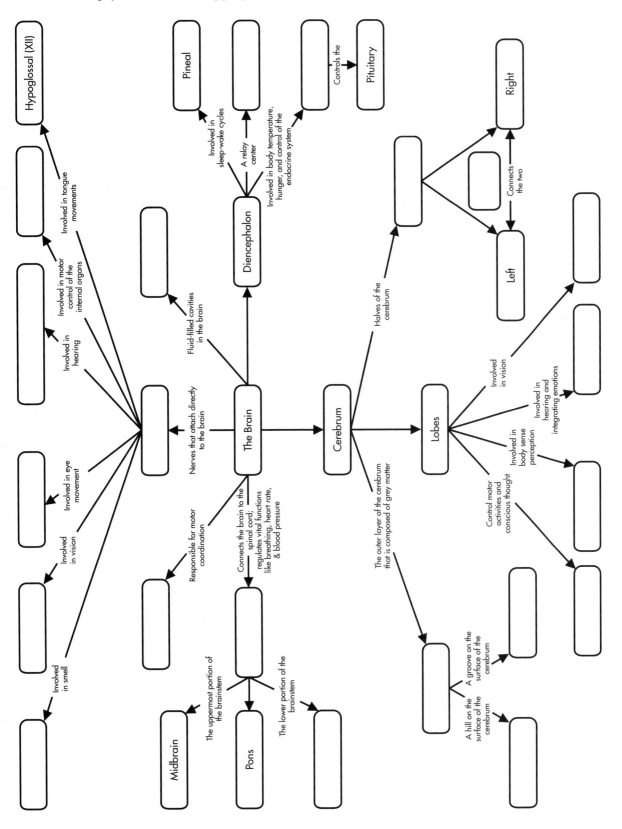

THE SENSES: THE SIGHTS AND SOUNDS

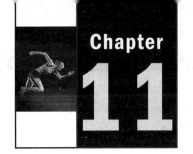

MEDICAL TERMINOLOGY REVIEW

Define the following terms.

1. Cataracts: _____
2. Presbyopia: _____
3. Myopia: _____
4. Amblyopia: _____
5. Glaucoma: _____
6. Vertigo: _____
7. Otitis media: _____
8. Labyrinthitis: _____
9. Phantom pain: _____
10. Referred pain: _____

MULTIPLE CHOICE

Circle the letter of the correct answer.

1. Which of the following correctly describes *phantom pain*?
    a. Pain at the location where a vital organ was recently removed
    b. Pain that originates in one part of the body but is felt in another
    c. Pain that is mysteriously felt in the daytime but is elusive at nighttime
    d. Pain or sensation felt in a limb that was amputated

2. Umami means:
    a. ringing in the ears.
    b. shadows in the visual spectrum.
    c. sporadic deafness and loss of equilibrium.
    d. taste of glutamates.

3. Which of the following is not a special sense?
    a. Sight
    b. Hearing
    c. Hunger
    d. Smell

Copyright © 2020 by Pearson Education, Inc.

4. How does the body rid itself of excess tears?
   a. The eyeball itself has the capacity to reabsorb the tears back into the aqueous humor
   b. With each and every blink, the eyelid collects the tears and directs them to the back of the orbit
   c. The face constricts its blood vessels, which increases the temperature of the eyeball and surrounding structures, and in turn evaporates the tears
   d. Excess tears drain into the nose via two small holes in the inner corner of the eye

5. Which of the following is true about the rods and cones?
   a. There are far more rods than cones.
   b. There are far more cones that rods.
   c. There are equal amounts of rods to cones.
   d. The number of rods and cones are correctable with prescription eyeglasses.

6. What is the primary function of the ossicles?
   a. Amplification of the sound waves that enter the middle ear
   b. Channeling of the sound waves that enter the outer ear
   c. Interpretation of sound waves that enter the inner ear
   d. to vibrate the ear drum

7. Which of the cranial nerves transmits from the cochlea and semicircular canals to the brain?
   a. Cranial nerve VIII
   b. Cranial nerve VI
   c. Abducens
   d. a and c

8. The eyeball sits in a conical cavity called the:
   a. Optic
   b. Orbit
   c. Ocular
   d. Olfactory

9. Which of these structures function as a sensor that activates a shielding effect as foreign objects approach the eyeball?
   a. Pupils
   b. Eyelashes
   c. Lens
   d. Eyebrows

10. Senses such as thirst, nausea, and the need to defecate are what kind of senses?
    a. Special
    b. Cutaneous
    c. Systemic
    d. Visceral

11. Which of the following is not a taste that the taste buds can detect?
    a. Sweet
    b. Spicy
    c. Bitter
    d. Sour

12. Where is the eardrum located?
    a. Between middle and inner ear
    b. Between the middle and outer ear
    c. Between the outer ear and labyrinth
    d. At the outer rim of the external auditory meatus

13. The sense of taste is referred to as:
    a. olfactory.
    b. gastration.
    c. mechanoreception.
    d. gustatory.

14. Arrange the ossicles in the direction that sound waves would travel through them.
    a. Malleus, incus, stapes
    b. Hammer, anvil, incus
    c. Stirrup, anvil, hammer
    d. Incus, malleus, stirrup

15. Which of the three layers of the eyeball is highly vascularized and also contains the iris?
    a. Cornea
    b. Choroid
    c. Retina
    d. Sclera

16. When there is low light, the iris will:
    a. defer activity to the rods.
    b. tighten.
    c. relax.
    d. rely on the cones.
17. The retina continues posteriorly to the back of the eye socket and forms what nerve?
    a. Oculomotor
    b. Optic
    c. Cranial nerve VIII
    d. b and c
18. The function of ear wax is to:
    a. filter sound.
    b. trap foreign particles.
    c. maintain surface tension of the inner ear.
    d. monitor pressure.
19. What is the function of the muscles surrounding the lens of the eye?
    a. To alter the shape of the lens, making it either thinner or thicker.
    b. To move the eyeball right, left, up, or down depending on the focal point
    c. To decrease or increase the diameter of the iris
    d. To push the lens forward or pull it back depending on the pressure of the fluids of the eye
20. When the iris contracts, what part of the eye changes, and in what way?
    a. Retina becomes wider
    b. Cornea becomes opaque
    c. Pupil becomes larger
    d. Pupil becomes smaller
21. Refinement of taste is primarily due to:
    a. location of receptor on tongue.
    b. sense of smell.
    c. memory.
    d. cravings.
22. Where are the olfactory receptors?
    a. Back of throat
    b. Roof of nasal cavity
    c. Sides of tongue
    d. In the organ of Corti
23. When Anne was 9 years old, she started having difficulty seeing the board from the back of the classroom. The teacher did not change the size of her script to warrant this gradual change in visual acuity. It was evident that Anne was the early stages of:
    a. myopia.
    b. glaucoma.
    c. otitis media.
    d. hyperopia.
24. Receptors of the skin, which include touch, heat, and pain, are referred to as:
    a. organ of Corti.
    b. visceral sense.
    c. cutaneous senses.
    d. dermatitis.
25. Sound travels best in:
    a. air at high altitudes.
    b. air at lower altitude.
    c. air at high temperature.
    d. solid or liquid medium.

MATCHING EXERCISES

Match each term with the appropriate definition.

Set 1

_____ 1. tympanic cavity
_____ 2. hammer
_____ 3. stirrup
_____ 4. pinna
_____ 5. anvil
_____ 6. cochlea
_____ 7. semicircular canals
_____ 8. endolymph
_____ 9. auditory tube
_____ 10. acoustic

a. canal or tube leading from the middle ear to the throat
b. middle ossicle between the malleus and the stapes
c. nerve also known as vestibulocochlear
d. auricle
e. fluid associated with organ of Corti
f. ossicle directly against the oval window
g. ossicle directly against the ear drum
h. cranial nerve VI
i. bony spiral structure of the inner ear associated with sound
j. another name for the middle ear
k. three canal loops of the inner ear associated more with equilibrium than actual sound

Set 2

_____ 1. myopia
_____ 2. labyrinthitis
_____ 3. tinnitus
_____ 4. conjunctivitis
_____ 5. otitis media
_____ 6. amblyopia
_____ 7. presbyopia
_____ 8. cataracts
_____ 9. glaucoma
_____ 10. hyperopia

a. lazy eye
b. inflammation of the lining of the eye
c. a ringing sound in the ears
d. inflammation of the inner ear
e. near sightedness
f. loss of taste
g. far sightedness
h. far sightedness brought about by age
i. infection of the middle ear
j. increased pressure in the fluid of the eye
k. clouded lens of the eye

Set 3

_____ 1. rods
_____ 2. cornea
_____ 3. cones
_____ 4. sclera
_____ 5. lens
_____ 6. pupil
_____ 7. lacrimal
_____ 8. vitreous
_____ 9. iris
_____ 10. aqueous

a. gland that secretes tears
b. humor that bathes the iris, pupil, and lens
c. bends light; surrounded by involuntary muscles
d. clinical term for the entire middle layer of the eyeball
e. sphincter that controls how much light passes into the eye
f. humor that occupies the posterior cavity of the eyeball
g. photoreceptors active in dim light
h. hole or circular opening in the middle of the sphincter muscle of the eyes
i. whites of the eye
j. photoreceptors active in bright light
k. transparent structure allowing outside light rays into the eye

Set 4

_____ 1. dermatome
_____ 2. adaptation
_____ 3. thermoreceptors
_____ 4. traction
_____ 5. olfactory receptors
_____ 6. pressure
_____ 7. tactile corpuscles
_____ 8. free nerve endings
_____ 9. PERRLA
_____ 10. papillae

a. temperature sensors
b. sensory receptors in the skin
c. neurological tests using the eye
d. area of skin innervated by one spinal nerve
e. located in roof of nasal cavity
f. a squeeze or pinch
g. contain receptors for sense of taste
h. a downward force
i. desensitization of sensory receptors due to repeated stimuli
j. nociceptors

FILL IN THE BLANK

Fill in the blanks to complete the following statements.

1. As it is associated with sound, the _____ of the inner ear sends sensory impulse to the _____ of the brain.
2. The inner ear is also called the _____.
3. Different people may have different pain _____, which affect perception of pain severity.
4. The glands that produce tears are the _____ glands.
5. Brown, hazel, blue, and green eyes are actually colors of the _____ of the eyeball.
6. The fluid that fills the posterior cavity of the eye is called _____.
7. The vibration of ossicles due to sound waves is _____ conduction.
8. The vestibule chamber of the ear houses the _____.
9. The part of the external ear that collects and directs sound waves into the external auditory meatus is the _____.
10. The ear drum is clinically called the _____ membrane.
11. The two fluids of the inner ear are the _____ and the _____.
12. The eustachian tube leads from the ear to the _____ of the throat.
13. As it is associated with equilibrium, the _____ of the inner ear sends sensory signals to the _____ of the brain.
14. Clouding of the lenses of the eyes is called _____.

15. Vision, hearing, and smell are known as _____ senses.
16. The medical term for pinkeye is _____.
17. _____ is tied closely to memory.
18. _____ and smell are closely related.
19. The sensations of pain, heat, thirst, and hunger are called _____ senses.
20. Ben recently turned 40 and had to start wearing glasses for the first time in his life. Without knowing anything else about him, what is the cause of his vision decrease? _____
21. _____ is the medical term for dizziness.
22. The body has more _____ receptors than receptors for any other sensation.
23. Ménière's disease affects the _____ of the ear.
24. Sensorineural hearing loss may result from damage to the _____.
25. Organ pain felt in another location is known as _____ pain.

SHORT ANSWER

1. Trace sound waves from their origin to your brain.
   _____
   _____
   _____
   _____

2. Explain the phenomenon called *adaptation* as it applies to sensation.
   _____
   _____
   _____
   _____

3. Describe the process of *accommodation* as it applies to the lens of the eye.
   _____
   _____
   _____
   _____

4. What are the three layers of the eyeball?

   _____
   _____
   _____
   _____

5. Contrast the three types of auditory conduction.

   _____
   _____
   _____
   _____

LEARNING ACTIVITIES

1. Your sense of taste is dependent on your sense of smell. Partner with a friend or group of friends. Using foods of similar texture (for example, potato and apple) test each other's abilities to identify food items solely based on taste. Try tasting the food while holding your nose. Can you identify the food?

2. The sense of touch is more sensitive on some parts of the body than on others. Explore this phenomenon using the "Two-Point Discrimination Test." Find a partner. To begin, one person should close his or her eyes while the other person gently touches two pins to the person's skin. Can the person tell that there are two pins? Move the pins closer together, then further apart. Next, test that person's ability to distinguish the pins on different parts of the body. Where can the pins be very close together? Where do they have to be further apart? Switch places and try the same test on the other partner.

3. Using a Snellen eye chart, test your visual acuity. If you wear corrective lenses, try it without your lenses.

4. Using the internet, research causes of blindness. What is the leading cause of blindness? What congenital or genetic disorders cause blindness?

112　　Chapter 11

 LABELING ACTIVITIES

1. Label the parts of the eye. Use Figure 11–2 in your textbook as a guide.

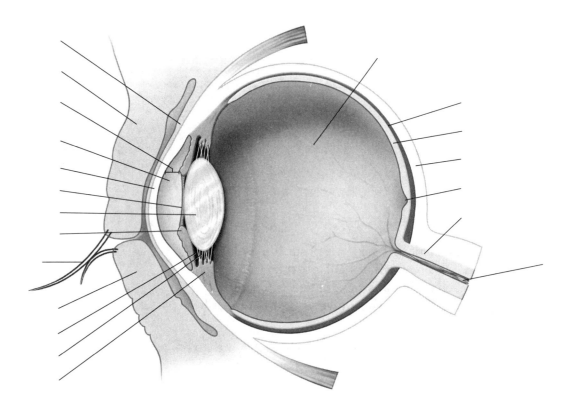

2. Label and color the parts of the ear. Use Figure 11–3 in your textbook as a guide.

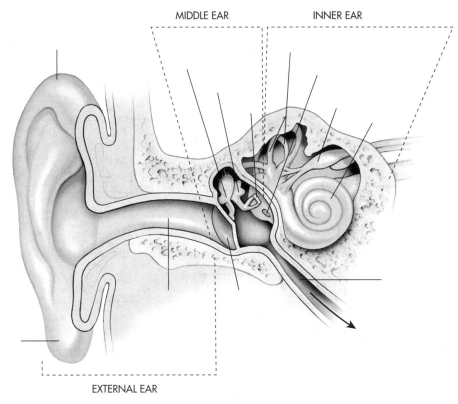

3. Label the referred pain map. Use Figure 11–9 in your textbook as a guide.

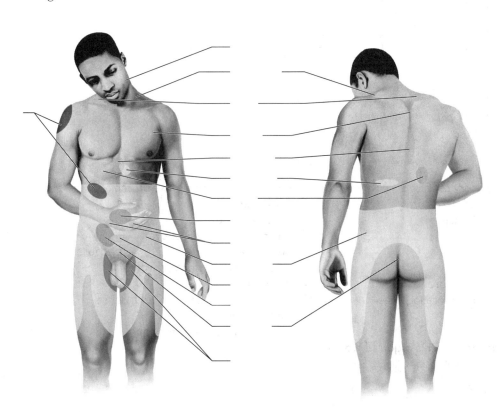

CROSSWORD PUZZLE

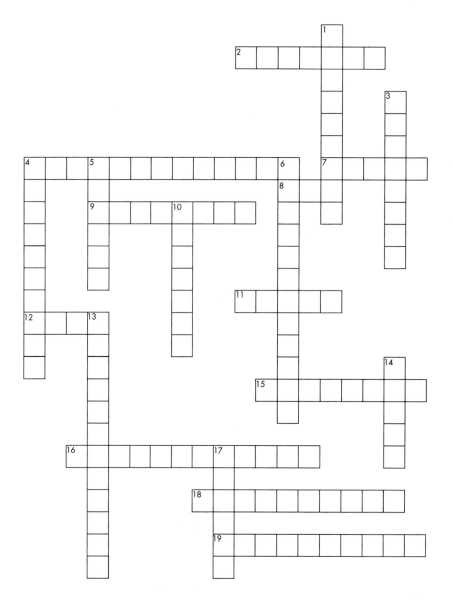

Across

2. structure containing sensory cells for hearing
4. _____ is the fluid filling the eyeball (2 words)
7. houses eyeball
8. organ of hearing
9. ear drum; _____ membrane
11. most important sense for interpreting taste
12. focuses light
15. ringing in the ears
16. auditory neurons embedded in this organ (3 words)
18. farsightedness associated with age
19. auditory or _____ tubes

Down

1. nerve which carries sense of smell
3. ear bones
4. balance sense
5. photoreceptor layer of eye
6. organ pain is _____ because it maps to body surface (2 words)
10. outer ear
13. _____ canals; vestibular sense
14. surrounds the iris
17. clear entrance to eye for light

Name _____

CONCEPT MAP

Fill in the empty boxes with an appropriate term using the clues provided.

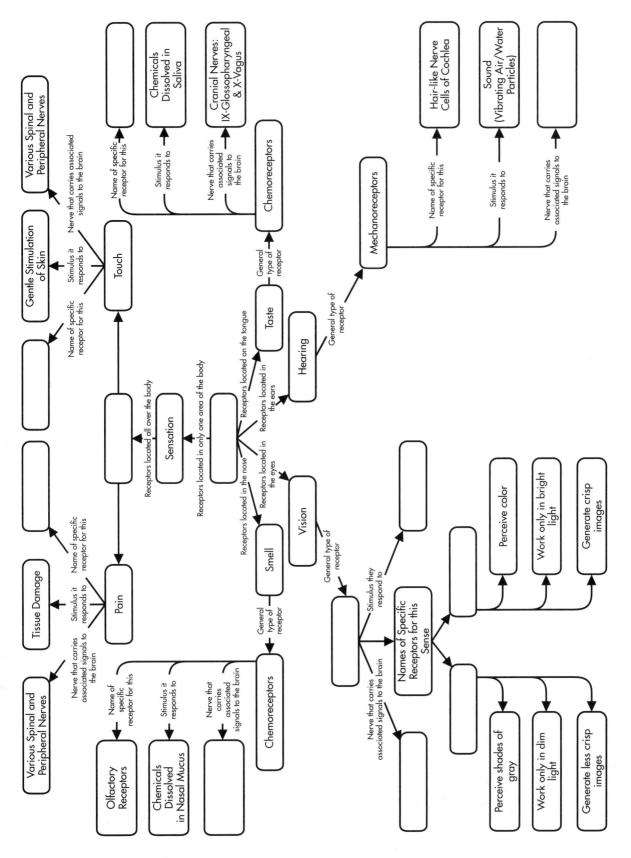

THE ENDOCRINE SYSTEM: THE BODY'S OTHER CONTROL CENTER

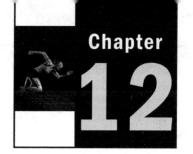

Chapter 12

MEDICAL TERMINOLOGY REVIEW

Define the following terms.
1. Hypothyroidism: _____
2. Hyperthyroidism: _____
3. Positive feedback: _____
4. Negative feedback: _____
5. Endocrine: _____
6. Hormone: _____
7. Steroids: _____
8. Cushing's syndrome: _____
9. Diabetes mellitus: _____
10. Goiter: _____

MULTIPLE CHOICE

Circle the letter of the correct answer.

1. What is the target organ(s) for glucagon?
   a. Pancreas
   b. Kidneys
   c. Adrenals
   d. Liver

2. How do hormones and neurotransmitters (NT) differ?
   a. Hormones are secreted by exocrine glands, and NTs are secreted from endocrine glands.
   b. Hormones are fast to take action, and NTs are slow to take effect.
   c. Hormones are secreted by endocrine glands, and NTs are secreted from axon terminals.
   d. b and c

3. Where are the adrenal glands located?
   a. Above the kidneys
   b. In the brain stem
   c. In the chest
   d. In the neck

4. On which feedback mechanism does insulin operate?
   a. Positive
   b. Negative
   c. Neutral
   d. Neural

5. Which hormone needs iodine for production?
   a. Insulin
   b. Thymosin
   c. Prolactin
   d. Thyroxine

6. Which gland or organ secretes releasing and inhibitory hormones controlling the master gland?
   a. Pituitary
   b. Adrenal
   c. Pancreas
   d. Hypothalamus

7. Where is the pancreas located?
   a. In the abdomen
   b. In the brain
   c. In the neck
   d. In the pelvis

8. What directly influences the production of testosterone?
   a. Gonadotropin-releasing hormone
   b. Corticotropic hormone
   c. Luteinizing hormone
   d. ACTH

9. What gland is at its greatest size and efficiency in childhood fighting infection and helping in the maturation of white blood cells?
   a. Thyroid
   b. Thymus
   c. Testis
   d. Adrenal

10. Which of the following is a function of one of the hormones secreted by the adrenal cortex?
    a. Fight or flight
    b. Salt and fluid balance
    c. Skin pigmentation
    d. Iodine production

11. What is the target organ for ACTH?
    a. Adrenals
    b. Adenoids
    c. Anterior pituitary
    d. Arterial walls

12. What is true about hormones?
    a. Focus on targets very close
    b. Affect a single cell
    c. Effects wear off quickly
    d. Effects are long lasting

13. Why are steroid hormones so powerful?
    a. Steroid hormones pass easily through the target cell membrane and interact with the cell's DNA.
    b. They are always secreted in great amounts.
    c. They interact with the neuronal cell bodies as well as the neural membranes.
    d. All of the above

14. What is the target organ for ADH?
    a. Adenoid
    b. Kidney
    c. Adrenal
    d. Pancreas

15. Which hormone antagonizes glucagon?
    a. Insulin
    b. Glycogen
    c. Thymosin
    d. Calcitonin

16. The control of blood sugar by pancreatic hormones is an example of this type of control.
    a. Hormonal
    b. Neural
    c. Glandular
    d. Humoral

17. What may occur if calcitonin is hypersecreted?
    a. Low blood calcium
    b. High blood cholesterols
    c. Low blood sugar
    d. High blood viscosity

18. Where is melanocyte-stimulating hormone produced?
    a. Posterior pituitary
    b. Thyroid
    c. Parathyroid
    d. Anterior pituitary

19. Which organ secretes a hormone but is not a primary endocrine organ?
    a. Pancreas
    b. Kidney
    c. Thyroid
    d. Pituitary

20. The diencephalon is home to the:
    a. hypothalamus.
    b. adrenals.
    c. thymus.
    d. pancreas.

21. Which hormone increases the release of LH and FSH from its releasing gland?
    a. Adrenocorticotropic hormone
    b. Estrogen
    c. Adrenocorticosteroids
    d. Gonadotropin releasing hormone

22. Parathyroid hormone targets the:
    a. bladder.
    b. skin.
    c. bone.
    d. mammary glands (breasts).

23. Polyuria (increased urination) is a symptom of:
    a. Addison's disease.
    b. diabetes mellitus.
    c. Cushing's syndrome.
    d. Hashimoto's disease.

24. For uterine contraction during childbirth the expectant mother needs to secrete:
    a. iodine.
    b. estrogen.
    c. oxytocin.
    d. prolactin.

25. A tumor of the adrenal gland resulting in excess secretion of epinephrine is called
    a. Hashimoto's disease.
    b. pheochromocytoma.
    c. Addison's disease.
    d. diabetes mellitus.

MATCHING EXERCISES

Match each term with the appropriate definition.

Set 1

_____ 1. pineal
_____ 2. anterior pituitary
_____ 3. posterior pituitary
_____ 4. ovaries
_____ 5. pancreas
_____ 6. thymus
_____ 7. testis
_____ 8. adrenal medulla
_____ 9. hypothalamus
_____ 10. thyroid

a. antidiuretic hormone
b. thyroxine
c. melanocyte-stimulating hormone
d. progesterone
e. testosterone
f. melatonin
g. insulin
h. thymosin
i. none
j. epinephrine

Set 2

_____ 1. parathyroid hormone
_____ 2. luteinizing hormone
_____ 3. follicle-stimulating hormone
_____ 4. triiodothyronine
_____ 5. oxytocin
_____ 6. calcitonin
_____ 7. insulin
_____ 8. norepinephrine
_____ 9. melatonin
_____ 10. adrenocorticosteroids

a. increases blood glucose
b. ovulation
c. decreases blood calcium
d. decreases blood sugar
e. regulates secondary sexual characteristics
f. increases blood calcium
g. increases metabolism; secreted by gland located in the neck
h. triggers sleep
i. milk ejection
j. prolongs fight-or-flight response
k. regulates sperm and egg production

Set 3

_____ 1. SIADH
_____ 2. Addison's disease
_____ 3. diabetes mellitus
_____ 4. dwarfism
_____ 5. bone deterioration
_____ 6. testicular shrinkage
_____ 7. Graves' disease
_____ 8. decreased milk production
_____ 9. impaired ovulation
_____ 10. Hashimoto's disease

a. steroid abuse
b. severe low blood sodium; overproduction of ADH
c. decrease in insulin production or recognition
d. hyposecretion of prolactin
e. swollen thyroid gland; hypothyroidism
f. decreased luteinizing hormone
g. decreased growth hormone during childhood
h. hypersecretion of parathyroid hormone
i. weight loss; low BP; insufficient cortisol
j. hyperthyroidism; bulging eyes

Set 4

_____ 1. pineal gland
_____ 2. anterior pituitary
_____ 3. posterior pituitary
_____ 4. ovaries
_____ 5. pancreas
_____ 6. thymus
_____ 7. testis
_____ 8. adrenal gland
_____ 9. hypothalamus
_____ 10. thyroid

a. in abdominal cavity
b. in diencephalon
c. external groin
d. near stomach
e. on kidney
f. attached to hypothalamus
g. posterior to thalamus
h. mediastinum
i. anterior neck
j. attached to diencephalon

FILL IN THE BLANK

Fill in the blanks to complete the following statements.

1. In females, _____ stimulates the smooth muscle tissue in the wall of uterus, promoting labor and delivery.
2. Another name for the anterior pituitary gland is _____.
3. The _____ is located in the mediastinum, posterior to the sternum.
4. The pancreas secretes _____ and _____.
5. A hyposecretion of cortisol causes _____.
6. T3 and T4 secretions are controlled by _____ secreted by the anterior pituitary.
7. Milk production is controlled by the hormone _____, and milk ejection is controlled by the hormone _____.
8. The hypothalamus regulates the release of hormones from the _____ gland.
9. FSH from the pituitary gland targets _____ and _____.
10. Alcohol inhibits the hormone _____.
11. The three ways hormone levels are regulated are _____, _____, and _____.
12. Prednisone (hydrocortisone) mimics the hormones secreted by the _____.
13. The antagonist hormone to calcitonin is secreted by the _____ gland.
14. _____ are chemical messengers that are released in one tissue and transported by the bloodstream to affect target cells and tissues.
15. The hormone unique to females is _____.
16. A(n) _____ is a tumor of the adrenal gland that causes excess epinephrine secretion.
17. Roberto is recovering from a serious head injury. Lately he has put on weight, his blood cholesterol and blood pressure are very high, and a recent minor injury is healing very slowly. What part of his brain might be damaged? _____
18. Overproduction of _____ may be involved with the pathological consequences of chronic stress.

19. Adults who secrete too much growth hormone have _____, whereas children who secrete too much growth hormone have _____.
20. The most common cause of _____ is Hashimoto's thyroiditis.
21. An enlargement of the thyroid called a(n) _____ can be caused by either hyperthyroidism or hypothyroidism.
22. Type 1 diabetes mellitus is caused by autoimmune destruction of the _____.
23. The body releases _____ several hours after a meal to prevent hypoglycemia.
24. _____ is stored in the liver and muscle cells and helps build protein.
25. _____ signaling occurs when a cell sends out a signal that affects nearby cells that are different from the cell sending out the signal.

SHORT ANSWER

1. Explain the functional difference between an exocrine gland and an endocrine gland.

2. What are two mutual side effects of anabolic steroid abuse in both men and women?

3. Why does alcohol increase urine output?

4. What is meant by *humoral* control of hormone levels?

5. Why are steroids and thyroid hormones particularly powerful?

LEARNING ACTIVITIES

1. For each hormone, list the effects on major systems. How many effects do you remember?
2. Using the internet, investigate the effects of anabolic steroids. Can you explain why the side effects happen given what you know about control of hormone levels?
3. Select one steroid hormone and do some research. What are the effects? How wide ranging are they?
4. Play "Name That Hormone." One student lists information about a hormone while other students try to identify the hormone. How many clues were needed?
5. Play "Endocrine System Twenty Questions." One student chooses a disease or an organ or a hormone. Other students ask questions requiring only "yes" or "no" answers to try to identify the term.

LABELING ACTIVITY

Name the pictured glands and list the primary function of each organ. Use Figure 5–11 in your textbook as a guide.

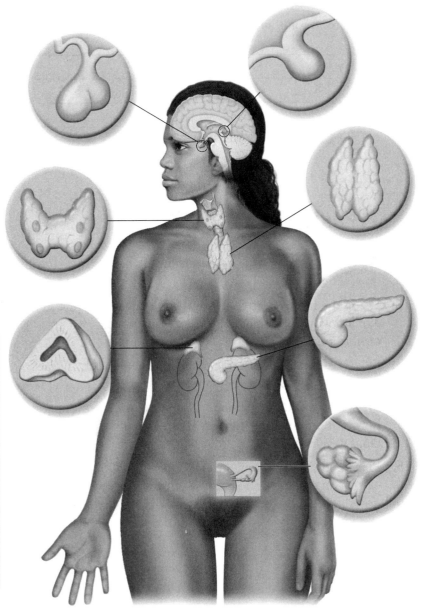

Organ	Primary Functions
Pituitary Gland	
Thyroid Gland	
Parathyroid Gland	
Thymus	
Adrenal Glands	
Pancreas	
Gonads	
Testes	
Ovaries	

Copyright © 2020 by Pearson Education, Inc.

CROSSWORD PUZZLE

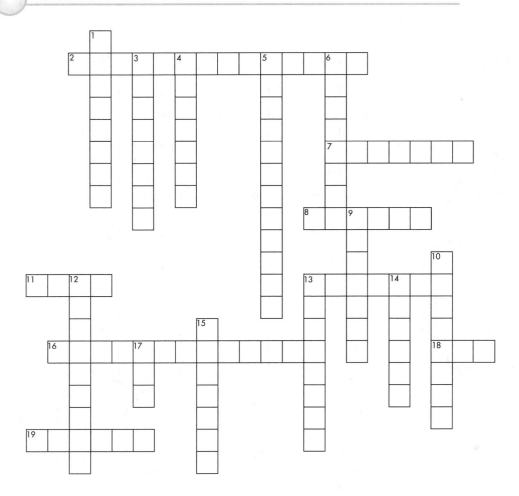

Across

2. sympathetic hormone
7. the _____ and parathyroid glands control calcium levels
8. secrete testosterone
11. stimulates adrenal cortex (abbreviation)
13. the _____ gland secretes steroid hormones
16. too little causes dwarfism (2 words)
18. abbreviation for hormone released from posterior pituitary
19. secretes melatonin

Down

1. stress hormone
3. released from ovaries
4. decreases blood sugar
5. controls pituitary gland
6. type of feedback involved in hormonal control
9. can cross cell membrane and interact directly with DNA
10. secreted when blood sugar drops
12. hormone that contains iodine
13. the _____ pituitary makes and secretes its own hormones
14. the release of epinephrine is under _____ control
15. chemical messenger released from endocrine glands
17. abbreviation for hormone that triggers release of T3 and T4

Name _____

CONCEPT MAP

Fill in the empty boxes with an appropriate term using the clues provided.

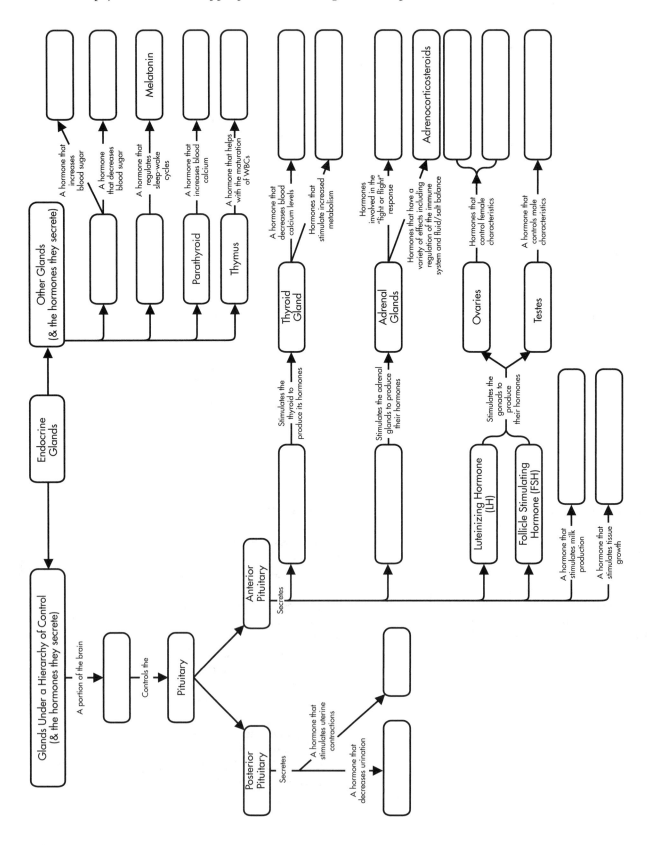

THE CARDIOVASCULAR SYSTEM: TRANSPORT AND SUPPLY

MEDICAL TERMINOLOGY REVIEW

Define the following terms.
1. Arteriosclerosis: _____
2. Thrombus: _____
3. Embolus: _____
4. Leukemia: _____
5. Myocardial infarct: _____
6. Ischemia: _____
7. Aneurysm: _____
8. Anemia: _____
9. Atherosclerosis: _____
10. Arrhythmia: _____

MULTIPLE CHOICE

Circle the letter of the correct answer.

1. The white blood cells that produce heparin are called:
   a. lymphocytes.
   b. basophils.
   c. eosinophils.
   d. erythrocytes.

2. The function of hemoglobin is:
   a. clotting.
   b. gas transport.
   c. immunity.
   d. production of blood cells.

3. Which of the blood types is considered the *universal recipient*?
   a. A
   b. O
   c. B
   d. AB

4. Where in the chest is the heart located?
   a. Directly in the middle of the chest, with apex above the base
   b. Slightly right of center with the base resting on the diaphragm
   c. Midline of chest, with the base directly resting on the diaphragm
   d. Slightly left of center with the base above the apex

Copyright © 2020 by Pearson Education, Inc.

5. Type B blood has _____ antigens and _____ antibodies.
   a. A, anti-B
   b. B, anti-A
   c. no, anti-A and anti-B
   d. A and B, no

6. The right side of the heart is responsible for:
   a. collecting and distributing oxygenated and deoxygenated blood to the right side of the body.
   b. collecting deoxygenated blood from all over the body and sending it just to the lungs.
   c. sending oxygenated blood to the upper body and collecting deoxygenated blood from the lower body.
   d. sending deoxygenated blood to and collecting oxygenated blood from the lungs.

7. Jose has type A blood. What type of blood can he receive in transfusion?
   a. B
   b. AB
   c. A
   d. All of the above

8. The left side of the heart is responsible for:
   a. collecting and distributing deoxygenated blood to the left side of the body.
   b. sending oxygenated blood to the lower body and collecting deoxygenated blood from the upper body.
   c. collecting oxygenated blood from the lungs and sending it to the entire body.
   d. sending deoxygenated blood to the lungs and collecting similar blood from the head.

9. Capillary walls are made of:
   a. simple squamous epithelium.
   b. smooth muscle.
   c. simple cuboidal epithelium.
   d. areolar tissue.

10. Which of the following is true of veins?
    a. Veins carry blood away from the heart.
    b. Veins have valves.
    c. Veins have thick tunica media.
    d. Veins always carry deoxygenated blood.

11. Which of the following explains cardiac output?
    a. A combination of blood flow and blood pressure
    b. Determined by heart rate and peripheral resistance
    c. Determined by heart rate and the amount of blood pumped with each contraction
    d. Determined by blood vessel diameter

12. What prevents blood from flowing into the left atrium upon ventricular contraction?
    a. The third chamber, called the atrioventricular chamber
    b. A valve called the tricuspid
    c. A valve called the mitral
    d. Decompression of the diaphragm

13. Which of the following is true with regard to the Rh factor?
    a. If an Rh-positive father and an Rh-negative mother have a child who inherits the father's blood type, it will be healthy, but the second child of the same couple will have complications if he or she is also Rh-positive
    b. If an Rh-negative father and an Rh-positive mother have a child who inherited the father's blood type, then there will be complications with the growth and development of this child
    c. If an Rh-positive father and an Rh-negative mother have a child who inherits the mother's blood type, it will be healthy, but their second child, if Rh-positive, will have complications
    d. If an Rh-positive father and an Rh-positive mother have an obvious Rh-positive child, it will be healthy, but their second child, if Rh-negative, will have complications

14. How does chewing an aspirin tablet help in a heart attack?
    a. Aspirin conducts electrical current that gives the heart muscles an instant jolt.
    b. Aspirin has the ability to vasoconstrict, temporarily raising blood pressure.
    c. Aspirin has anticoagulating ability to help blood flow easier.
    d. Aspirin increases RBCs, allowing more oxygen to the heart muscles.

15. As fluid volume increases, what happens to blood pressure?
    a. It rises.
    b. It falls.
    c. It stays the same.
    d. There is no relationship between fluid volume and BP.

16. Which of the following statements is true?
    a. The right ventricle sends blood to both the right and left lungs to pick up a fresh supply of oxygen.
    b. The left ventricle sends blood to both the right and left lungs to pick up a fresh supply of oxygen.
    c. The right ventricle sends blood to the right lung, and the left ventricle sends blood to the left lung to pick up a fresh supply of oxygen.
    d. The right and left atria direct blood to the right and left lungs, respectively.

17. Which of the walls of the heart chambers is the thickest?
    a. Atrioventricular
    b. Left ventricle
    c. Right atria
    d. Left atria

18. Which of the following is an influence on blood pressure?
    a. Heart rate
    b. Blood vessel diameter
    c. Blood volume
    d. All of the above

19. Correctly arrange the electrical wiring of the heart from where the impulse is initially generated to where it is carried to the muscle cells.
    a. Bundle of His, vagus nerve, sino-atrial node, atrioventricular node
    b. Sino-atrial node, vagus nerve, Purkinje cells, atrioventricular node, bundle of His
    c. Sino-atrial node, atrioventricular node, bundle of His, Purkinje fibers
    d. Vagus nerve, sino-atrial node, atrioventricular node, Purkinje fibers, bundle of His

20. On the ECG, which of the waves represents the depolarization of the atria?
    a. T
    b. QRS
    c. It is masked by another wave
    d. P

21. What happens in the last stage of coagulation?
    a. Soluble fibrinogen is converted to insoluble fibrin.
    b. A platelet plug is formed.
    c. Platelets are activated.
    d. Prothrombin is converted to thrombin.

22. What happens immediately after the depolarization of the ventricles?
    a. The atria contract.
    b. The atria relax.
    c. The ventricles contract.
    d. The ventricles relax.

23. How much blood do humans normally have?
    a. 1 to 3 liters
    b. 4 to 6 liters
    c. 7 to 9 liters
    d. 11 to 13 liters

24. What is the function of hemoglobin?
    a. Clots blood
    b. Carries oxygen
    c. Threads a biological net
    d. Keeps blood from clotting

25. Sympathetic output to the _____ affects blood pressure.
    a. SA node
    b. tunica media
    c. myocardium
    d. All of the above

MATCHING EXERCISES

Match each term with the appropriate definition.

Set 1

_____ 1. monocytes
_____ 2. phagocytosis
_____ 3. erythrocytes
_____ 4. basophils
_____ 5. leukocytes
_____ 6. lymphocytes
_____ 7. erythropoiesis
_____ 8. neutrophils
_____ 9. thrombocytes
_____ 10. eosinophils

a. produce antibodies
b. the process by which RBCs are created
c. a granulocyte that attempts to destroy bacteria by engulfing
d. WBCs involved in allergies and inflammation
e. WBCs functioning to combat parasites and decrease allergies
f. the process by which a cell surrounds and ingests an invader
g. collective term for white blood cells
h. collective term for red blood cells
i. higher than normal amounts in chronic infections
j. platelets

Set 2

_____ 1. agglutination
_____ 2. pallor
_____ 3. tunic
_____ 4. embolus
_____ 5. inotropism
_____ 6. node
_____ 7. anastomoses
_____ 8. vasoconstriction
_____ 9. vasodilation
_____ 10. iron

a. arterial reaction resulting in increased pressure within the vessel
b. deficiency may lead to anemia
c. pale skin
d. self-antigens on RBC cell surface bind to antibodies, clumping
e. branching of arteries so there is ample blood supply to the entire heart
f. a layer of a blood vessel
g. results in increased blood vessel diameter
h. pacemaker
i. traveling clot
j. means the force of cardiac contractions
k. mineral produced by the heart

Set 3

_____ 1. hemophilia
_____ 2. cerebral vascular accident
_____ 3. left-side heart failure
_____ 4. anemia
_____ 5. aneurysm
_____ 6. myocardial infarction
_____ 7. atherosclerosis
_____ 8. arteriosclerosis
_____ 9. leukemia
_____ 10. valvular insufficiency

a. blood backs up into lungs causing pulmonary edema
b. accumulation of plaque in vessels
c. the mitral valve may be too large
d. high amounts of immature WBCs
e. hardening of the blood vessels
f. uncontrollable bleeding
g. low amount of viable RBCs
h. weakening of arterial wall
i. heart attack
j. stroke

Set 4

_____ 1. sinoatrial node
_____ 2. vagus nerve
_____ 3. calcium
_____ 4. medulla oblongata
_____ 5. clotting factors
_____ 6. antidiuretic hormone
_____ 7. norepinephrine
_____ 8. acetylcholine
_____ 9. serotonin
_____ 10. fever

a. releases neurotransmitter to decrease heart rate
b. neurotransmitter that increases peripheral resistance
c. proteins necessary for coagulation
d. increases fluid volume
e. constricts smooth muscle and decreases blood flow
f. heart pacemaker
g. neurotransmitter that decreases heart rate
h. increased concentration can prolong heart condition
i. increases heart rate and blood pressure
j. contains vital centers for control of heart rate and blood pressure

FILL IN THE BLANK

Fill in the blanks to complete the following statements.

1. Arteries move blood _____ the heart.
2. The wall that separates the two lower chambers of the heart is called the _____.
3. On the ECG, the wave that represents the depolarization of the ventricles is the _____.
4. Blood transports _____, _____, _____ and _____.
5. Upon separation by centrifugation, blood is seen to have two major components: _____ and _____.
6. In the clotting mechanism, prothrombin, produced by the _____, is converted to thrombin with the help of vitamin _____.
7. The wall that separates the two upper chambers of the heart is called the _____.

8. Blood from the right upper chamber drains through the _____ valve to the lower chamber on the same side.

9. When body temperature increases, the response of the cardiac rate and force is to _____.

10. The SA node is located in/on the _____ of the heart.

11. The electrolyte _____, when at high levels, can prolong heart contractions to the point that the heart can actually stop beating.

12. The biological "net" or "gauze" made of _____ is formed by posttrauma attempts to cover the wound and prevent blood cells from escaping.

13. When examining the plaque removed from a blood vessel, you will find the main component of this substance is _____.

14. Two instruments, the _____ and the _____, are used to determine a patient's or client's blood pressure.

15. The two large vessels that empty into the right atrium are the _____ and the _____.

16. A blood pressure reading in the range of 130–139 over 85–89 is classified as _____.

17. Buildup of plaque in blood vessels leading to reduce blood flow is known as _____.

18. _____ (hardening of the arteries) leads to brittle, less flexible blood vessels.

19. Rapid, uncoordinated contractions of heart muscle are called _____.

20. Jerry prides himself on being in excellent physical condition, but lately he has not felt well. He is tired all the time and has no energy. His friends have also noticed he is extremely pale. Thinking it might be his diet, he adds more leafy greens and occasional red meat to his diet. He feels much better. What is Jerry's condition? _____

21. Lori is a competitive runner. While in graduate school she lived and trained in western Colorado. Now that she is living and training on the coast, she notices that her endurance seems to have decreased. She had more endurance previously due to _____, thanks to the high altitude.

22. The _____ deliver oxygenated blood to body tissues and take away carbon dioxide.

23. A floating clot is called a(n) _____.

24. A weak spot in the wall of an artery that could rupture and cause a massive hemorrhage is called a(n) _____.

25. Mike wakes his wife in the middle of the night because he is not feeling well. He is nauseous and dizzy. His left shoulder aches and he is having trouble catching his breath. What is most likely happening to Mike? _____

SHORT ANSWER

1. Contrast the terms *agglutination* and *coagulation*.

2. Explain the exception to the rule that arteries carry oxygenated blood and veins carry deoxygenated blood.

3. Explain blood flow through the heart.

4. Explain the control of blood pressure.

5. Explain how heart valves work.

LEARNING ACTIVITIES

1. There are several types of leukemia classified by the type of cells involved. Using the internet, research the various types of this disease. What cells are involved for each type? Is the prognosis different for each type?

2. In 1986, a volleyball player named Flo Hyman died during a game. Her death was attributed to a ruptured aortic aneurysm due to Marfan's syndrome, a connective tissue disorder. Using the internet or any other source, find out how Marfan's syndrome causes aneurysms.

3. Draw the cardiovascular system on a large piece of paper and divide it into squares, similar to a board game. Make a set of cards with questions on them. Every third space should have a symbol indicating that players must answer a question. If a player cannot answer the question, he or she must give up his or her next turn. The object of the game is to get from the right atrium through pulmonary and systemic circulation and back to the right ventricle. Make some cards worth extra places. Use dice to determine how many spaces should be moved each turn.

4. Using a model of the heart, or a preserved heart, identify each of the parts. Using a pencil or probe, and trace blood flow through the heart.

5. Play "Cardiovascular Disorder Twenty Questions." One student chooses a cardiovascular disorder and other students may ask up to 20 yes or no questions in an attempt to guess the disorder.

LABELING ACTIVITY

Label the figure and color the blood vessels using red to indicate oxygenated blood, blue to indicate deoxygenated blood, and purple to indicate where the oxygen level changes. Use Figure 13–1 in your textbook as a guide.

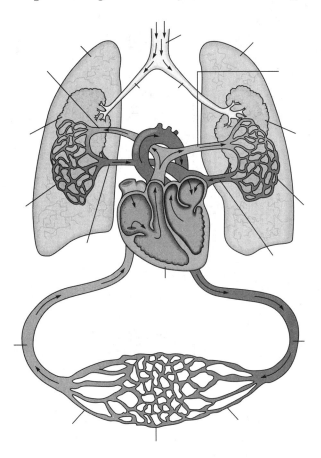

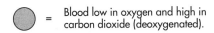 = Blood low in oxygen and high in carbon dioxide (deoxygenated).

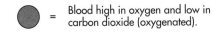 = Blood high in oxygen and low in carbon dioxide (oxygenated).

CROSSWORD PUZZLE

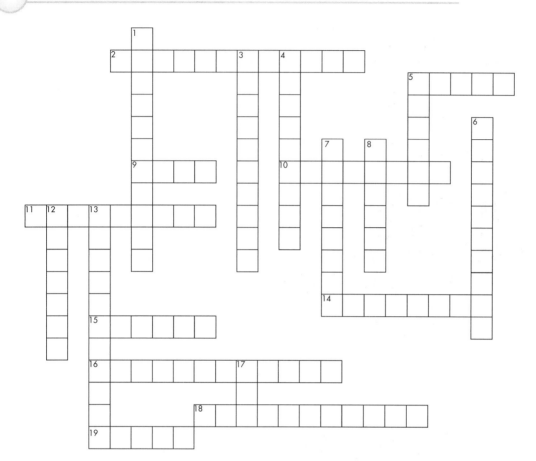

Across

2. decreases peripheral resistance
5. the vessel that carries blood from the left ventrical
9. arteries carry blood _____ from the heart
10. a narrowing of a valve is called _____
11. cardiac cycle refers to contraction of this chamber
14. impulse spreads from AV node to _____ (2 words)
15. superior vena cava empties into the right _____
16. red blood cells
18. clotting
19. type A blood has these antibodies (2 words)

Down

1. smallest blood vessels
3. technical term for white blood cells
4. the valve between the right atrium and ventricle
5. can be caused by decreased hemoglobin or RBCs
6. soluble fiber in platelet plug
7. cancer which results in large numbers of white blood cells
8. ADH controls BP by controlling blood _____
12. floating blood clot
13. layer of blood vessel innervated by sympathetic axons (2 words)
17. stroke abbreviation

Name _____

CONCEPT MAP

Fill in the empty boxes with an appropriate term using the clues provided.

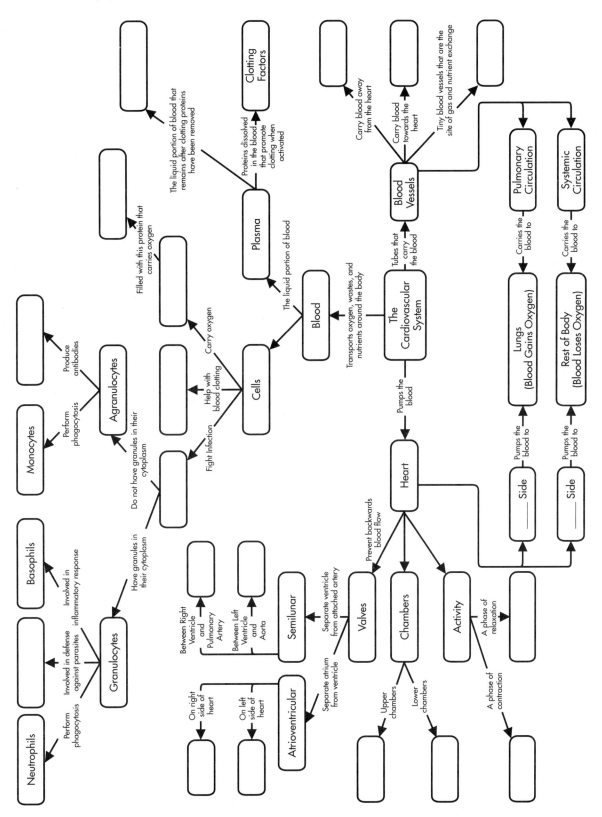

THE RESPIRATORY SYSTEM: IT'S A GAS

Chapter 14

MEDICAL TERMINOLOGY REVIEW

Define the following terms.
1. Atelectasis: _____
2. Emphysema: _____
3. Tuberculosis: _____
4. Pneumothorax: _____
5. Asthma: _____
6. Ventilation: _____
7. Respiration: _____
8. Chronic obstructive pulmonary disease: _____
9. Pleural effusion: _____
10. Tidal volume: _____

MULTIPLE CHOICE

Circle the letter of the correct answer.

1. What type of cells make up the membrane that lines the respiratory region of the nose and most of the airway?
   a. Stratified ciliated cuboidal
   b. Simple squamous
   c. Stratified ciliated squamous
   d. Pseudostratified ciliated columnar

2. The region that separates one lung from the other is called:
   a. pleura.
   b. mediastinum.
   c. carina.
   d. septum.

3. The purpose of pleural fluid is to:
   a. reduce friction as an individual breathes.
   b. moisten air passages.
   c. filter debris.
   d. reduce surface tension within the bronchioles.

4. The main function of surfactant is to:
   a. nourish the trachea.
   b. reduce friction as a person swallows.
   c. reduce surface tension in the alveoli.
   d. filter gases in the nasal cavity.

Copyright © 2020 by Pearson Education, Inc.

5. Which of the following statements is/are true about sinuses?
   a. They connect to the nasal cavity via small passageways.
   b. Humans are born with three of the four sinuses.
   c. The sinuses are filled with air, making the skull heavier and more protective.
   d. All of the above

6. Which of the three sections of the pharynx contains the adenoids?
   a. Tracheopharynx
   b. Nasopharynx
   c. Oropharynx
   d. Laryngopharynx

7. Which of the following statements is true about inspiration?
   a. For inspiration to take place, pressure in the thoracic cavity needs to decrease
   b. For inspiration to take place, atmospheric pressure needs to be lower than thoracic pressure
   c. For inspiration to take place, pressure in the thoracic cavity needs to increase
   d. For inspiration to take place, atmospheric pressure and thoracic pressure need to be equal

8. What is the purpose of cilia in the airways?
   a. To propel air into the lungs
   b. To propel trapped debris upward to be expelled from the body
   c. To trap food and prevent entry into the windpipe
   d. To aid in olfaction

9. Which of the three sections of the pharynx conducts air, food, and liquid?
   a. Oropharynx
   b. Nasopharynx
   c. Tracheopharynx
   d. All of the above

10. The lobes of the lungs are subdivided into _____ with one bronchus in each subdivision.
    a. lobules
    b. bronchioles
    c. alveoli
    d. segments

11. Which of the paired tonsils is located in the middle pharyngeal section?
    a. Adenoid
    b. Palatine
    c. Lingual
    d. Submandibular

12. Directly below the Adam's apple is a large cartilage called the:
    a. thyroid cartilage.
    b. epiglottic cartilage.
    c. arytenoid cartilage.
    d. cricoid cartilage.

13. How does the epiglottis work during swallowing?
    a. As we breathe in, the epiglottis moves from its natural closed position to an open position so air can enter the larynx and trachea.
    b. As we swallow, the epiglottis flaps down to close off the larynx so food does not slip into that area.
    c. As we breathe in, the epiglottis closes off our esophagus so air does not enter into that area.
    d. It acts as a "guard gate," closing off the eustachian tubes so air and food cannot enter and cause problems.

14. The name of the membrane that covers or wraps each lung is:
    a. pulmonary sheath.
    b. synovial membrane.
    c. visceral pleura.
    d. parietal aponeurosis.

15. The function of the conchae is to:
    a. warm and moisten air.
    b. filter large particles.
    c. trap oxygen so it remains in the airways.
    d. prevent the entrance of carbon dioxide into the airways.

16. There are two _____ bronchi.
    a. primary
    b. segmental
    c. lobular
    d. respiratory

17. Inert gas, in the context of the respiratory system, means it:
    a. is poisonous to the continuation of life.
    b. does not combine or interact in the body.
    c. is necessary for sustaining life.
    d. is depleting slowly from the atmosphere.

18. The process of gas exchange in which carbon dioxide is removed from the blood and oxygen is added is called:
    a. internal respiration.
    b. internal ventilation.
    c. external respiration.
    d. external ventilation.

19. Arrange the following gases from highest to lowest percent in the atmosphere.
    a. Oxygen, carbon dioxide, nitrogen, argon
    b. Nitrogen, oxygen, carbon dioxide, argon
    c. Oxygen, carbon dioxide, argon, nitrogen
    d. Carbon dioxide, hydrogen, oxygen, argon

20. Which of the following is not part of the respiratory membrane?
    a. Alveolar epithelium
    b. Capillary epithelium
    c. Interstitial space
    d. Smooth muscle of the alveolar duct

21. Where does the upper airway or upper respiratory tract end?
    a. Just below the nasopharynx
    b. Just below the vocal cords
    c. Just below the trachea
    d. Just behind the nasal cavity

22. Which of the following is true of the walls of the tracheobronchial tree as air moves from the trachea to the alveoli?
    a. Epithelium changes from pseudostratified to simple squamous
    b. The amount of cartilage increases
    c. The amount of smooth muscle increases
    d. Epithelium changes from simple cuboidal to stratified squamous

23. The bulk movement of air down to the lungs is termed:
    a. ventilation.
    b. respiration.
    c. transgasideous migration.
    d. pulmonary peristalsis.

24. Where is the olfactory region of the nose?
    a. Behind the nostril to the sides of the cartilage
    b. Against the septum of the nasal cavity
    c. At the rear of the nasal cavity on the tops of the uvula and soft palate
    d. On the roof of the nasal cavity

25. Which of the following is not a function of the upper airway?
    a. Heating and cooling of inspired air
    b. Phonation
    c. Olfaction
    d. External respiration

MATCHING EXERCISES

Match each term with the appropriate definition.

Set 1

_____ 1. rectus abdominis
_____ 2. external intercostals
_____ 3. vibrissae
_____ 4. vertebrocostal
_____ 5. glottis
_____ 6. medulla oblongata
_____ 7. turbinates
_____ 8. vertebrosternal
_____ 9. sternum
_____ 10. carina

a. receptor(s) of smell
b. conchae
c. nose hair
d. true ribs
e. breastbone
f. contain(s) the vocal cords
g. muscle of expiration
h. respiratory control center
i. muscle of inspiration
j. where the trachea ends and primary bronchi begins
k. false ribs

Set 2

_____ 1. capillary endothelium
_____ 2. squamous pneumocytes
_____ 3. terminal bronchiole
_____ 4. alveolar epithelium
_____ 5. interstitial
_____ 6. pores of Kohn
_____ 7. macrophages
_____ 8. surfactant
_____ 9. respiratory bronchioles
_____ 10. granular pneumocytes

a. coats the inner most layer of the alveoli
b. marks the end of the conducting area of the lower respiratory tract
c. lead to the alveolar ducts
d. allow type III cells to move from one alveolus to another
e. make up the majority of the actual tissue layer of the alveolus
f. ingest foreign particles as they wander through the alveoli
g. produce a phospholipid substance that acts on surface tension
h. layer of respiratory membrane that is nearest to blood
i. space that separates the alveoli from the capillaries
j. the actual tissue layer of the air sac functional units
k. substance that increases surface tension

Set 3

_____ 1. pneumonia
_____ 2. tuberculosis
_____ 3. emphysema
_____ 4. hydrothorax
_____ 5. erythropoietin
_____ 6. asthma
_____ 7. pneumothorax
_____ 8. atelectasis
_____ 9. hemoglobin
_____ 10. hemothorax

a. molecule that carries large amounts of oxygen
b. constriction of the airway in response to an allergy
c. clinical term for the influenza virus
d. infectious disease; vast lung damage can occur
e. lung infection; inflammation with accumulation of cell debris and fluid
f. blood in the pleural space
g. when the air sacs of the lungs are partially or totally collapsed
h. air in the thoracic cavity
i. hormone that influences RBC production
j. irreversible condition in which air sacs become destroyed
k. fluid accumulation in the pleural space

Set 4

_____ 1. tidal volume
_____ 2. residual volume
_____ 3. inspiratory reserve
_____ 4. expiratory reserve
_____ 5. inspiratory capacity
_____ 6. functional residual capacity
_____ 7. vital capacity
_____ 8. total lung capacity
_____ 9. pulmonary capacities
_____ 10. pulmonary volumes

a. inspiratory reserve + tidal volume + expiratory reserve
b. ventilation volumes that are actually measured
c. ventilation volumes that are calculated
d. air inspired forcefully after normal inspiration
e. volume of air moved during a normal inspiration
f. expiratory reserve vol. + residual vol.
g. air forcefully expired after normal expiration
h. air left in lungs after maximum expiration
i. tidal vol. + inspiratory reserve vol.
j. inspiratory reserve + expiratory reserve + tidal vol. + residual vol.

FILL IN THE BLANK

Fill in the blanks to complete the following statements.

1. The mechanism involving mucus and cilia that removes debris from airways is known as the _____ escalator.
2. The three sections of the pharynx are the _____, the _____, and the _____.
3. The voice box is clinically known as the _____.
4. The common name for the trachea is the _____.
5. The part of the tracheobronchial tree in which there is no gas exchange is known as the _____ zone.
6. The region of the lung called the _____ is where pulmonary arteries exit, pulmonary veins enter, and the main stem of the bronchus can be found entering the lung.

7. The prime muscle of inspiration is called the _____.
8. The right lung has _____ lobes and the left lung has _____ lobes.
9. A substance called surfactant can be found in the _____.
10. Both men and women have _____ pairs of ribs, _____ of which are true ribs and _____ are floating ribs.
11. Located just above the clavicle is the _____ of the lungs.
12. When thoracic volume increases, the thoracic pressure _____.
13. The gas exchange surface of the lung is/are the _____.
14. When exercising or participating in strenuous work, the depth of breathing _____ and the rate of breathing _____.
15. The eustachian tubes lead from the _____ to the _____.
16. The motor neurons for the respiratory system are located in this part of the brain: _____.
17. _____ is the gas that controls ventilation rate and depth.
18. Receptors in the _____ measure blood chemistry and control ventilation rate.
19. The primary etiology for COPD, except asthma, is _____.
20. Inhaled foreign bodies more often end up in which lung? _____
21. The _____ nerve innervates the diaphragm.
22. Sierra fell off her bicycle while riding. Initially, she felt fine, but today she is having trouble catching her breath and is coughing. Upon examination she has a large bruise on her chest and reduced breath sounds. Her lung has _____.
23. Gwen smoked for years. Recently, she has developed breathing difficulty. Tests reveal no masses or fluid, but her alveoli are greatly expanded. What is the diagnosis? _____
24. You lose your voice after screaming at a concert, causing inflammation. What is this disorder called? _____
25. In the actual gas exchange areas of the lungs there is no _____ because it would decrease gas exchange.

SHORT ANSWER

1. Explain the mechanism of inspiration.

2. What are the primary functions of the respiratory system?

3. Besides the diaphragm, what muscles play a role in inspiration? How do they aid inspiration?

4. Contrast internal and external respiration.

5. How is blood chemistry related to ventilation?

LEARNING ACTIVITIES

1. Use a balloon to demonstrate the relationship of volume to pressure changes. Fill the balloon with air. Squeeze the balloon to lower the volume. Eventually, the balloon will pop. Did the pressure increase inside the balloon as you decreased the volume by squeezing or did it decrease? What would happen if you could somehow make the balloon bigger without adding air? Try the same thing with the bulb of a turkey baster. Squeeze the air out. As you stop squeezing and allow the bulb to expand (increasing the volume), what happens to pressure inside the bulb? Does air flow into the bulb or out?

2. Cigarette smoking causes a number of respiratory disorders. Use the internet to research the possible long-term effects of cigarette smoking. How many disorders are linked to smoking?

3. Each part of the respiratory system has a unique function. For each part, list that function and one disorder that interferes with that function.

4. Make a set of flashcards with the name of a part of the respiratory system on one side and either the anatomy or function on the other. Quiz your partner.

5. Design a respiratory system board game. Draw the upper and lower airways and lungs. Each space should be associated with a question about a specific part of the respiratory system. Each player is an oxygen molecule. The object is to get from the atmosphere to the blood. Roll dice to determine how many spaces can be moved. Answering the question correctly allows movement on the board.

LABELING ACTIVITY

Label the various structures of the respiratory system. Use Figure 14–1 in your textbook as a guide.

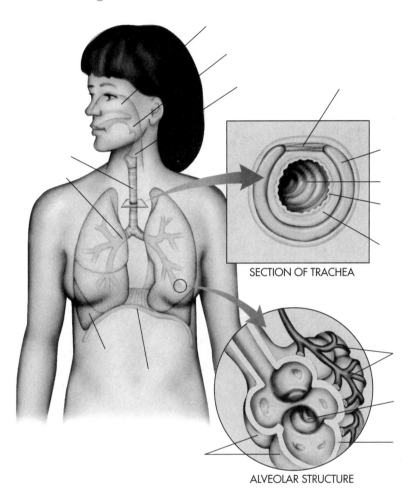

SECTION OF TRACHEA

ALVEOLAR STRUCTURE

CROSSWORD PUZZLE

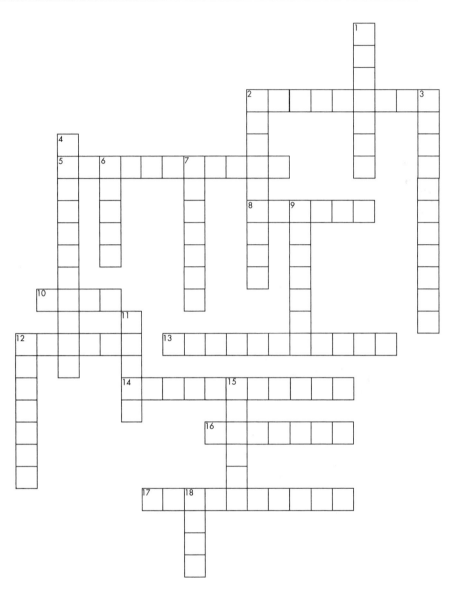

Across

2. the prime muscle of inspiration
5. zone of tracheobronchial tree where gas exchange occurs
8. breathing difficulty often triggered by allergies
10. group of disorders including emphysema and chronic bronchitis (abbreviation)
12. serous membrane in thoracic cavity
13. bulk movement of air into and out of respiratory system
14. collapse of alveoli
16. lobar _____, one in each lobe of each lung
17. may be missing or decreased in premature babies

Down

1. Adam's apple; _____ cartilage
2. when the diaphragm contracts, thoracic pressure _____
3. _____ escalator; cilia moving mucus
4. small airways
6. cavity in facial bone, connected to nasal cavity
7. air sacs
9. wind pipe
11. cavity posterior to nose
12. motor nerve for diaphragm
15. split of trachea into main bronchi
18. 12 pairs, part of thoracic cage

Name _____

CONCEPT MAP

Fill in the empty boxes with an appropriate term using the clues provided.

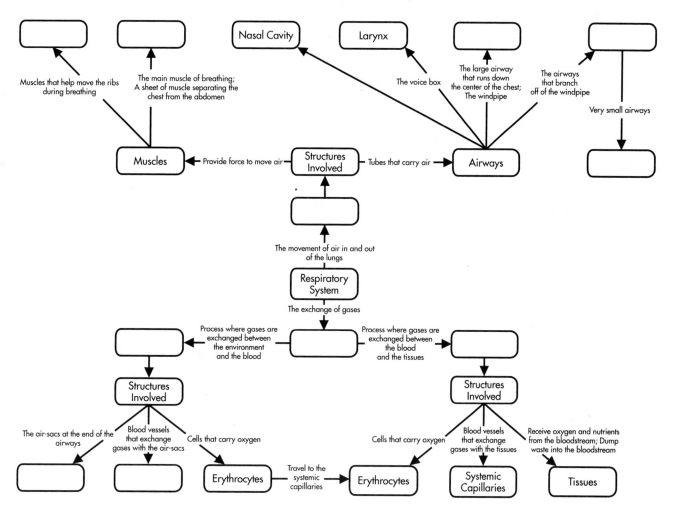

THE LYMPHATIC AND IMMUNE SYSTEMS: YOUR DEFENSE SYSTEMS

Chapter 15

MEDICAL TERMINOLOGY REVIEW

Define the following terms.

1. Anaphylaxis: _____
2. Cytokine: _____
3. Antibody: _____
4. Antigen: _____
5. Acquired immune deficiency syndrome: _____
6. Autoimmune disorder: _____
7. Innate immunity: _____
8. Adaptive immunity: _____
9. Lymph node: _____
10. Leukemia: _____

MULTIPLE CHOICE

Circle the letter of the correct answer.

1. Which stage of cancer is often terminal?
   a. 4
   b. 3
   c. 2
   d. 1

2. Physical barriers of the immune system include:
   a. skin.
   b. mucous membranes.
   c. saliva.
   d. All of the above

3. How do antibodies destroy pathogens?
   a. May cause the antigens to clump
   b. Pinocytosis
   c. Exocytosis
   d. Pull the antigen to the body surface, ulcerate the skin, and then release the antigen to the external environment

4. What do the lymphatic system, innate immunity, and adaptive immunity have in common?
   a. Rid the body of invading pathogens
   b. Lie dormant until needed
   c. Never turn on themselves
   d. Get stronger and better with age

5. After the physical barriers, which of the following is considered the first line of defense in the body?
   a. Antibodies
   b. Histamines
   c. Heparin
   d. Phagocytosis

6. The function of the spleen is to:
   a. produce red blood cells.
   b. differentiate T lymphocytes.
   c. help WBCs mature.
   d. filter pathogens from the bloodstream.

7. The right lymphatic duct empties into the:
   a. thoracic duct.
   b. jugular vein.
   c. subclavian vein.
   d. spleen.

8. How does lymph move through the body?
   a. Body movement
   b. Heart
   c. Gravity
   d. Centrifugal force

9. Lymphatic trunks empty into:
   a. collecting ducts.
   b. subclavian veins.
   c. lymph nodes.
   d. thymus.

10. Where is the spleen located?
    a. Between the heart and the sternum
    b. Upper right quadrant of abdomen
    c. Upper left quadrant of pelvis
    d. Upper left quadrant of abdomen

11. Which of the following areas have large concentrations of lymph nodes?
    a. Lumbar
    b. Subclavian
    c. Inguinal
    d. All of the above

12. Where do lymphocytes originate?
    a. Yellow bone marrow
    b. Red bone marrow
    c. Spleen
    d. Lymph nodes

13. Which one of the WBCs does the human immunodeficiency virus specifically target?
    a. Helper B cells
    b. Helper T cells
    c. Plasma cells
    d. Macrophages

14. Antibodies passed on to a fetus through the placenta represent:
    a. innate immunity.
    b. naturally acquired passive immunity.
    c. artificially acquired passive immunity.
    d. naturally acquired active immunity.

15. These cells release a chemical, perforin, that destroys pathogens or infected cells.
    a. Natural killer cells
    b. Plasma cells
    c. Dendritic cells
    d. Cytotoxic T cells

16. A vaccine is an example of:
    a. innate immunity.
    b. artificially acquired active immunity.
    c. artificially acquired passive immunity.
    d. naturally acquired active immunity.

17. What is the role of antigen-presenting cells?
    a. Repel pathogens
    b. Activate helper T cells
    c. Flag cells for destruction
    d. All of the above

18. Inflammation is often thought of as a two-edged sword. Why?
    a. Too much inflammation can suppress the immune system
    b. Too much inflammation encourages infection
    c. Too much inflammation causes leukemia
    d. Too much inflammation causes tissue damage

19. Which WBC is the first to arrive at the site of damage?
    a. Macrophage
    b. Plasma cell
    c. Neutrophil
    d. Lymphocyte

20. Increase in body temperature due to infection represents:
    a. innate immunity.
    b. naturally acquired passive immunity.
    c. artificially acquired passive immunity.
    d. naturally acquired active immunity.

21. How does innate immunity enhance adaptive immunity?
    a. Antigen-presenting cells
    b. Release of cytokines
    c. Complement
    d. All of the above

22. Autoimmune disorders may result from the failure of these cells:
    a. cytotoxic T cells.
    b. regulatory T cells.
    c. memory T cells.
    d. helper T cells.

23. Which of the following is an effect of activation of complement cascade?
    a. Inflammation
    b. T cell activation
    c. B cell activation
    d. Enhanced phagocytosis

24. Survival and activation of lymphocytes that recognize self-antigens is called:
    a. positive selection.
    b. autoimmunity.
    c. negative selection.
    d. allergies.

25. Which of the following is true about the function of the thymus gland?
    a. It has a higher functioning capacity in children than in adults.
    b. It contains lymphocytes.
    c. It secretes a hormone.
    d. All of the above

MATCHING EXERCISES

Match each term with the appropriate definition.

Set 1

_____ 1. leukocyte
_____ 2. neutrophil
_____ 3. interferon
_____ 4. macrophage
_____ 5. basophil
_____ 6. eosinophil
_____ 7. natural killer cells
_____ 8. dendritic cell
_____ 9. cytotoxic
_____ 10. plasma cells

a. phagocytic granulocytes; most common WBC
b. releases chemicals to promote inflammation
c. all-encompassing term for white blood cells
d. adaptive immunity T-lymphocyte
e. cytokine that protects neighboring cells from viral attack
f. phagocytic modified monocytes; innate immunity
g. produce antibodies
h. counteracts activity of basophils; active during parasitic infections
i. modified monocytes acting as antigen-presenting cells
j. innate lymphocytes that secrete chemicals to kill cells displaying antigens

Set 2

_____ 1. primary immune response
_____ 2. secondary immune response
_____ 3. cell-mediated immunity
_____ 4. turn off immune response
_____ 5. natural active immunity
_____ 6. artificial passive immunity
_____ 7. artificial active immunity
_____ 8. natural passive immunity
_____ 9. innate immunity
_____ 10. tumor necrosis factor inhibitor

a. memory B cells
b. plasma cell
c. perforin
d. regulatory T cells
e. treats rheumatoid arthritis
f. physical barrier
g. the flu shot
h. accidentally exposed to a pathogen like chicken pox
i. being injected with antibodies
j. breast milk

Set 3

_____ 1. memory cells
_____ 2. histamines
_____ 3. interleukin-1
_____ 4. lymph
_____ 5. antigens
_____ 6. fungi
_____ 7. radiation
_____ 8. venoms
_____ 9. interleukin-2
_____ 10. antibodies

a. secreted by helper T cells
b. located on cell surface
c. remembers pathogens
d. secreted by macrophages
e. pathogenic organism
f. inflammation-causing physical agent
g. inflammation-causing chemical agent
h. secreted by mast cells
i. carries antigens to nodes around the body
j. secreted by the plasma cells

Set 4

_____ 1. leukemia
_____ 2. cancer
_____ 3. rheumatoid arthritis
_____ 4. HIV/AIDS
_____ 5. SCID
_____ 6. allergies
_____ 7. lupus erythematosis
_____ 8. type 1 diabetes
_____ 9. anaphylaxis
_____ 10. asthma

a. autoimmune attack on synovial membrane
b. immune response to harmless antigen
c. autoimmune destruction of many different tissues
d. destruction of helper T cells by virus
e. abnormal cells spread into lymphatic system
f. autoimmune destruction of pancreatic cells
g. respiratory distress triggered by allergies
h. cancer causing excess production of leukocytes
i. systemic immune response, causes widespread vasodilation
j. genetic immune deficiency

FILL IN THE BLANK

Fill in the blanks to complete the following statements.

1. When your body mounts a hyperactive response to a harmless antigen, the reaction is called a(n) _____.
2. The lymphatic tissue inside the lymph nodes contains _____ and _____.
3. The survival of competent lymphocytes is known as _____.
4. Helper T cells are also called _____ cells.
5. In order to fight off thousands of pathogens, lymphocytes must make thousands of copies of themselves. This process is called lymphocyte _____.
6. A hypersensitivity reaction called _____ leads to _____ blood pressure and heart failure.
7. List one effect of inflammation that makes it useful: _____.
8. _____ cells are attacked by the HIV virus.
9. When cancer has spread to nearby lymph nodes, it is in stage _____.
10. The destruction of lymphocytes that recognize and bind to the body's antigens is called _____.
11. The lymphatic tissue inside a lymph node is surrounded by _____.
12. During an allergic reaction, pollen directly activates the release of _____.
13. Redness, swelling, heat, and possible pain are all _____ symptoms.
14. B cells and cytoxic T cells are activated by _____.
15. Interferon and interleukins are both chemicals collectively called _____.
16. _____ are stimulated to divide by binding to antigen-presenting cells.
17. During the maturation process, _____ become differentiated.
18. The three sets of tonsils include the _____, _____, and _____.
19. _____ is a cytokine that stimulates macrophages and kills cancer cells.
20. A series of chemical reactions that activate more than 20 proteins is called _____ _____.

21. Memory cells mediate _____ response.
22. Decreased immune function is also called _____.
23. Macrophages, monocytes, and several other types of phagocytic cells found in organs and tissues are part of the _____ system.
24. List one physical barrier: _____.
25. _____ drugs suppress the immune system.

SHORT ANSWER

1. Besides through viruses such as HIV that causes AIDS, how can a patient's immune system become compromised?
   _____
   _____
   _____
   _____

2. What is the primary function of lymph nodes?
   _____
   _____
   _____
   _____

3. Structurally contrast the spleen and large lymph nodes.
   _____
   _____
   _____
   _____

4. Explain the connections between innate and adaptive immunity.
   _____
   _____
   _____
   _____

5. Why are CD-4 cells so important?
   _____
   _____
   _____
   _____

LEARNING ACTIVITIES

1. Create a series of flash cards for each part of the immune system with the component on one side and the function on the other.

2. You are the immune system. Flu viruses have invaded your body. What do you do? List the steps taken by the immune system to fight off the virus.

3. Patients with suppressed immune systems often develop opportunistic infections. What is an opportunistic infection? List the common opportunistic infections found in patients whose immune systems are compromised.

4. Play "Immune System Twenty Questions."

5. For each part of the immune system, come up with an analogy not found in the book. The book used warfare and fire departments. Can you think of other analogies?

158 Chapter 15

  LABELING ACTIVITY

In the box provided, list the functions of each part of the lymphatic system and label the identified structures. Use Figure 5–14 in your textbook as a guide.

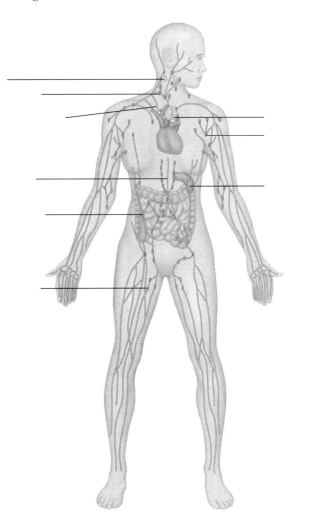

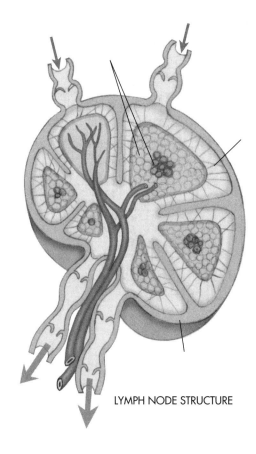

LYMPH NODE STRUCTURE

Copyright © 2020 by Pearson Education, Inc.

CROSSWORD PUZZLE

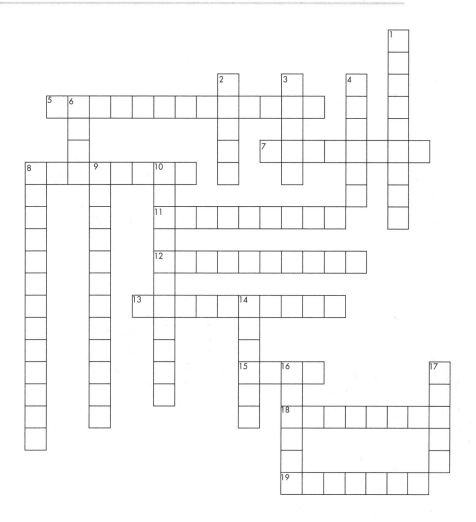

Across

5. _____ cells: the only lymphocytes in innate immunity (2 words)
7. chemical released by T cells for direct cell killing
8. selection for immune competent lymphocytes
11. _____ T cell; cell mediated immunity
12. protects cells from viral infection
13. antigen displaying cell
15. one of the body's physical barriers
18. selection against lymphocytes which react to self-antigens
19. antibodies and complement _____ phagocytosis

Down

1. chemicals which enhance immunity
2. skin response to hypersensitivity reaction
3. increased body temperature
4. _____ B cells mediate secondary response
6. full blown disorder caused by HIV
8. reproduction of activated lymphocytes
9. swelling, heat, redness, pain
10. deliberate exposure of patient to weakened or dead pathogen
14. B cell responsible for primary response
16. inborn, does not recognize specific pathogens
17. helper, cytotoxic, memory and regulatory for example (2 words)

Name _____

CONCEPT MAP

Fill in the empty boxes with an appropriate term using the clues provided.

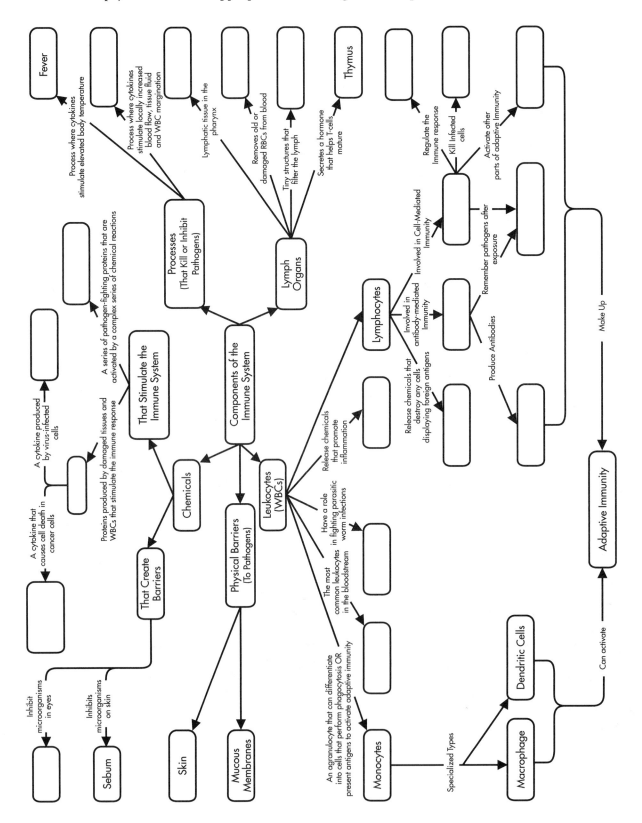

THE GASTROINTESTINAL SYSTEM: FUEL FOR THE TRIP

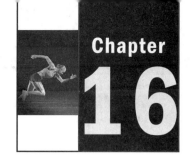

MEDICAL TERMINOLOGY REVIEW

Define the following terms.
1. Cholecystitis: _____
2. Pancreatitis: _____
3. Hepatitis: _____
4. Diverticulitis: _____
5. Gastroesophageal reflux disease: _____
6. Caries: _____
7. Cirrhosis: _____
8. Gastroenteritis: _____
9. Peptic ulcer: _____
10. Ulcerative colitis: _____

MULTIPLE CHOICE

Circle the letter of the correct answer.

1. Which of the salivary glands is located under the tongue?
   a. Parotid
   b. Submandibular
   c. Sublingual
   d. Palatial

2. If not pulled or knocked out, how many permanent teeth do people have by 25 years of age?
   a. 32
   b. 16
   c. 28
   d. 42

3. Please arrange the segments of the large intestine in the order waste travels through.
   a. Cecum, descending colon, ascending colon, transverse colon, sigmoid colon, rectum
   b. Cecum, ascending colon, transverse colon, descending colon, sigmoid colon, rectum
   c. Sigmoid colon, ascending colon, transverse colon, descending colon, cecum, rectum
   d. Sigmoid colon, descending colon, ascending colon, transverse colon, cecum, rectum

4. When food enters the mouth it is said to be:
   a. ingested.
   b. digested.
   c. absorbed.
   d. All of the above

5. The digestive enzyme secreted by the pancreas that digests proteins is called:
   a. peptidase.
   b. amylase.
   c. pepsin.
   d. cholecystokinin.

6. Where does 80 percent of absorption of usable nutrients take place?
   a. Stomach
   b. Mouth
   c. Large intestine
   d. Small intestine

7. Which nerve innervates the visceral muscles of the stomach, causing contraction and hence motility?
   a. Phrenic
   b. Vagus
   c. Trigeminal
   d. Sciatic

8. The *labia* is/are commonly known as the:
   a. tongue.
   b. gallbladder.
   c. lips.
   d. uvula.

9. What does *emulsify* mean in terms of fat?
   a. The building of fatty acid chains in the liver
   b. The binding of fatty acids to carrier proteins for transport to the liver
   c. The destruction of fat globules or the rendering of fat globules unusable so no absorption will ever take place
   d. The breaking or converting of fat into a form that promotes enzymatic chemical digestion

10. Which sphincter lies between the stomach and small intestine?
    a. Cardiac
    b. Gastroenteral
    c. Pyloric
    d. Ileocecal

11. What is the pH of HCl in the stomach?
    a. 1.5 to 2.0
    b. 7.0 to 7.2
    c. 7.5 to 8.8
    d. 12.0 to 13.6

12. What is the function of the liver?
    a. Detoxification
    b. Production of clotting factors
    c. Storage of glucose in a form called glycogen
    d. All of the above

13. What is a *lacteal*, and where is it located?
    a. Lymphatic capillary in each villus of small intestine
    b. Blood capillary beside goblet cells in the pancreas
    c. Enzyme in the pancreas that, when secreted, digests milk
    d. Mucous lining found in the stomach

14. In the stomach, what do the parietal cells secrete, and what do the chief cells secrete?
    a. Sucrose/fructose
    b. Amylase/lipase
    c. HCl/pepsinogen
    d. Bile/bilirubin

15. In reference to the cardiac sphincter, where is the fundus of the stomach?
    a. Left, superior
    b. Right, inferior
    c. Left, inferior
    d. Right, superior

16. What structure prevents people from swallowing their tongues and also aids in proper speaking?
    a. Diaphragm
    b. Uvula
    c. Epiglottis
    d. Frenulum

17. Which section of the small intestine connects to or is continuous with the stomach?
    a. Cecum
    b. Duodenum
    c. Ileum
    d. Jejunum

18. Which of the following statements is correct?
    a. The hepatic ducts conduct bile from the liver, the cystic duct conducts bile to and from the gallbladder, and the common bile duct conducts bile to the small intestine.
    b. The common bile duct conducts bile from the liver, the cystic duct conducts bile to and from the gallbladder, and the hepatic ducts conduct bile to the small intestine.
    c. The cystic duct conducts bile from the liver, the hepatic ducts conduct bile to and from the gallbladder, and the common bile duct conducts bile to the small intestine.
    d. The common bile duct conducts bile from the liver, the hepatic ducts conduct bile to and from the gallbladder, and the cystic duct conducts bile to the small intestine.

19. Where is the most common region for peptic ulcer disease?
    a. Distal and middle parts of the esophagus
    b. Body of the stomach
    c. Upper or proximal part of small intestine
    d. Rectum and around the anal sphincter

20. The vermiform appendix hangs off the:
    a. cecum.
    b. rectum.
    c. colon.
    d. ileum.

21. What effect does secretin have on the stomach?
    a. Increases muscular activity
    b. Produces bile
    c. Increases secretions
    d. Decreases overall activity

22. How many incisors do adults normally have?
    a. 4
    b. 6
    c. 8
    d. 10

23. The uvula is associated with which structure?
    a. Soft palate
    b. Hard palate
    c. Tongue
    d. Pharynx

24. What substance starts chemically breaking down in the mouth due to salivary secretions?
    a. Starch
    b. Protein
    c. Fat
    d. Lactose

25. Bilirubin from what is eliminated in bile?
    a. Fat
    b. Food
    c. Feces
    d. Blood cells

MATCHING EXERCISES

Match each term with the appropriate definition.

Set 1

_____ 1. cirrhosis
_____ 2. enteritis
_____ 3. polyposis
_____ 4. calculi
_____ 5. hemorrhoids
_____ 6. Crohn's disease
_____ 7. gingivitis
_____ 8. gastritis
_____ 9. volvulus
_____ 10. cholecystitis

a. twisting of the bowel that causes obstruction
b. inflammation of the stomach
c. chronic disease of the liver
d. inflammation of the gallbladder
e. constipation or fecal impacting at the transverse colon
f. regional ileitis
g. inflammation of the small intestine
h. small tumors found in the colon
i. inflammation of the gums
j. varicose veins of the rectum
k. gall stones

Set 2

_____ 1. secretin
_____ 2. cholecystokinin
_____ 3. pepsin
_____ 4. hydrochloric acid
_____ 5. bile
_____ 6. peptidase
_____ 7. intrinsic factor
_____ 8. gastrin
_____ 9. sucrase
_____ 10. amylase

a. breaks down protein in stomach
b. emulsifies fat
c. breaks down starches in mouth
d. neutralizes the chyme in duodenum
e. needed for the absorption of B_{12}
f. stimulates the release of bile
g. breaks down dissaccharides
h. breaks down protein in small intestine
i. hormone that increases gastric activity
j. digests portions of protein structures of small intestine
k. converts pepsinogen to pepsin
l. hormone that activates bile production

Set 3

_____ 1. chyle
_____ 2. rugae
_____ 3. gingival
_____ 4. Peyer's patch
_____ 5. adventitia
_____ 6. villi
_____ 7. epiglottis
_____ 8. nitroglycerine
_____ 9. cementum
_____ 10. bolus

a. medication used to increase gastric juices
b. folds in the stomach
c. anchors root of tooth to gums
d. lymph tissue in small intestine
e. food stuff mixed with salivary juices
f. food stuff mixed with gastric juices
g. finger like protrusions in small intestine
h. absorbable under the tongue
i. gum
j. outer layer of the esophagus
k. prevents food from slipping into lungs
l. lipoproteins in the lacteal formed from glycerol and fatty acids

Copyright © 2020 by Pearson Education, Inc.

Set 4

_____ 1. esophagus
_____ 2. stomach
_____ 3. small intestine
_____ 4. large intestine
_____ 5. oral cavity
_____ 6. gallbladder
_____ 7. liver
_____ 8. pancreas
_____ 9. salivary gland
_____ 10. appendix

a. may replenish beneficial bacteria in digestive tract
b. most digestion and absorption
c. release digestive enzymes into duodenum
d. begins starch digestion and mechanical breakdown of food
e. secretes enzyme that digests starch
f. stores bile
g. makes bile
h. makes and stores feces
i. transports food to stomach, no digestion
j. stores food, digests protein

FILL IN THE BLANK

Fill in the blanks to complete the following statements.

1. Any organ whose function and size seem to have been reduced as humans evolved is termed _____.
2. Another name for canine teeth is _____.
3. Gastric activities, such as churning and secretion of enzymes, are controlled by the _____ nervous system (be specific).
4. For most of the digestive tract, the serosa layer is also called _____.
5. Between the ages of 2 and 3, all _____ of your baby teeth should have appeared.
6. The clinical term for the elimination of unusable material from the body is _____.
7. The digestive tract is also called the _____ tract.
8. If fecal material moves through the large intestine too fast, _____ occurs.
9. The _____ protects the airway during swallowing.
10. The three main regions of the large intestine are the _____, _____, and _____.
11. Besides food from the stomach, the first part of the small intestine receives additional secretions from the _____ and the _____.
12. Baby teeth are clinically called _____ teeth.
13. Heartburn occurs when the _____ opens and there is a backflow of food.
14. The digestive enzyme found in saliva is _____.

15. If fecal material moves too slowly through the intestine, _____ occurs.
16. People who cannot digest dairy products are _____ intolerant.
17. The treatment for appendicitis is a(n) _____, removal of the appendix.
18. _____ are varicose veins in the anus.
19. One function of the _____ is to detoxify the body of harmful substances.
20. Inflammation of the gallbladder may lead to inflammation of this nearby accessory organ _____.
21. A protrusion of the stomach through the diaphragm and into the thoracic cavity is called a(n) _____ _____.
22. _____, a yellowish tinge to the skin, is one symptom of liver disease.
23. Two common symptoms of digestive illness are _____ and _____.
24. The duodenum is a _____ organ because it is covered in parietal peritoneum rather than visceral.
25. The cephalic phase of gastric secretion begins when you _____ food.

SHORT ANSWER

1. What is the purpose of villi, plicae circulares, and microvilli in the small intestine?

   _____
   _____
   _____
   _____

2. Explain the three phases of gastric secretion.

   _____
   _____
   _____
   _____

3. List the functions of the liver.
   _____
   _____
   _____
   _____

4. List the digestive hormones and their functions.
   _____
   _____
   _____
   _____

5. List the accessory organs and their functions.
   _____
   _____
   _____
   _____

LEARNING ACTIVITIES

1. For each part of the digestive system, list the function.
2. Design a digestive system board game. Draw the alimentary canal and accessory organs. Each space should be associated with a question about a specific part of the digestive system. Each player is food. The object is to get from the plate to the anus. Roll dice to determine how many spaces can be moved. Answering the question correctly allows movement on the board.
3. List the symptoms for each of the major digestive disorders. How similar are they? How can you make an accurate diagnosis?
4. Diet has a great deal of influence on digestive health. List the kinds of foods that often cause trouble. Which disorders are obviously influenced by food choices?
5. Colorectal cancer is a common cancer in the United States. Do some research on this disease. What is the screening test? Why are polyps important? How can colorectal cancer be prevented? How can it be treated?

LABELING ACTIVITY

Label the organs and structures in the figure. Use Figure 16-1 in your textbook as a guide.

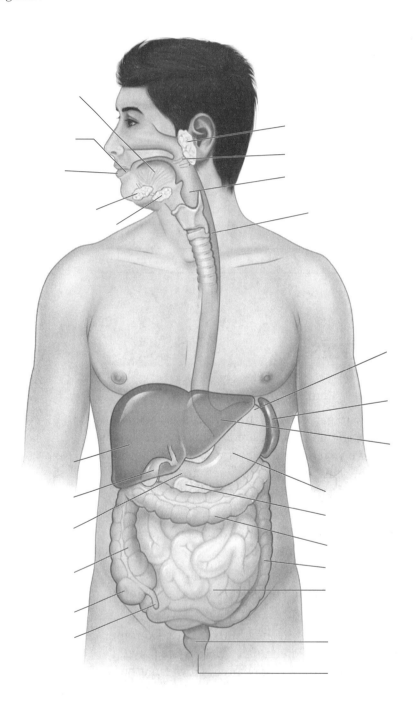

CROSSWORD PUZZLE

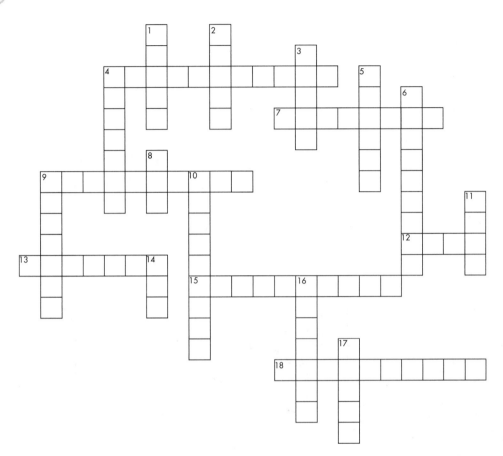

Across

4. stores bile
7. phase of gastric activity that begins before you even eat
9. valves between parts of alimentary canal
12. starch is digested in this cavity
13. part of stomach connected to esophagus
15. small intestine does almost all of this
18. serous membrane lining abdominal cavity

Down

1. medical term for large intestine
2. projections that increase surface area of small intestine
3. stored in large intestine
4. increases stomach activity
5. digested by amylase
6. breakdown of food into nutrients
8. acid in stomach (abbreviation)
9. stores food
10. no digestion takes place here
11. emulsifier
14. decreases stomach activity (abbreviation)
16. digestion begins in stomach
17. detoxification organ

Name _____

CONCEPT MAP

Fill in the empty boxes with an appropriate term using the clues provided.

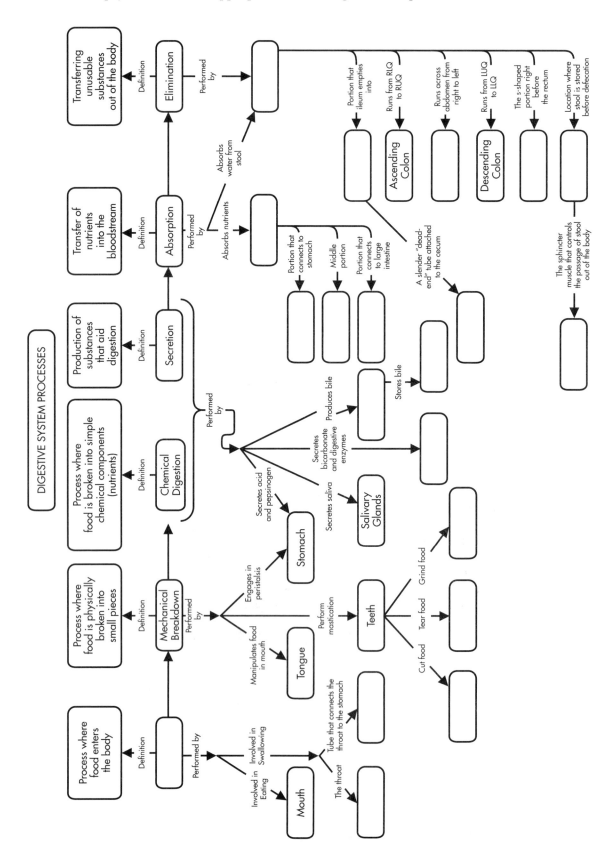

THE URINARY SYSTEM: FILTRATION AND FLUID BALANCE

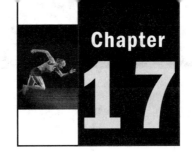

MEDICAL TERMINOLOGY REVIEW

Define the following terms.
1. Polycystic kidney disease: _____
2. Diabetic nephropathy: _____
3. Glomerulonephritis: _____
4. Glomerulosclerosis: _____
5. Analgesic nephropathy: _____
6. Lithotripsy: _____
7. Renal failure: _____
8. Ischemia: _____
9. Creatinine: _____
10. Antidiuretic hormone: _____

MULTIPLE CHOICE

Circle the letter of the correct answer.

1. The renal capsule covers the:
   a. kidney.
   b. glomerulus.
   c. bladder.
   d. afferent arteriole.

2. Which of the following will not pass through the glomerular epithelium into the nephron?
   a. RBC
   b. WBC
   c. Protein molecules
   d. All of the above

3. Glucose is _____ in glomerular filtrate than in urine.
   a. at the same concentration
   b. at a higher concentration
   c. at a lower concentration
   d. none of the above

4. The urinary bladder walls are composed of what type of muscle(s)?
   a. Smooth
   b. Voluntary
   c. Skeletal
   d. b and c

5. One of the symptoms of kidney stones is:
   a. pale urine.
   b. blood in urine.
   c. lower back numbness.
   d. excessive, uncontrollable, painless urination with continual expulsion of crystalline structures.

6. Urea is _____ in plasma than in urine.
   a. at the same concentration
   b. at a higher concentration
   c. at a lower concentration
   d. none of the above

7. Besides water, which of the following substances is usually found in urine at the bladder level?
   a. Glucose
   b. Ammonia
   c. Protein
   d. All of the above

8. Where are the kidneys located?
   a. Upper abdomen
   b. Lower abdomen
   c. Scrotal sac
   d. Pelvic cavity

9. Which of these urinary organs transports urine from the kidneys to the bladder?
   a. Nephrons
   b. Urethra
   c. Ureter
   d. Glomerulus

10. Urea and creatinine are _____ in urine than in glomerular filtrate.
    a. at the same concentration
    b. at a higher concentration
    c. at a lower concentration
    d. none of the above

11. Sodium is _____ in plasma then in urine.
    a. at the same concentration
    b. at a higher concentration
    c. at a lower concentration
    d. none of the above

12. In which layer of the kidney is blood filtered?
    a. Pelvis
    b. Medulla
    c. Cortex
    d. Capsule

13. Which of the following structures is located in the renal medulla?
    a. Major calyces
    b. Pyramids
    c. Glomerulus
    d. Minor calyces

14. Normally, how can humans consciously control the expulsion of urine from the body?
    a. Conscious control over the urinary bladder muscle
    b. Conscious control over the ureter sphincters
    c. Conscious control over the urethral sphincters
    d. Conscious control over the production of urine

15. Which of the following is the correct order in which blood arrives at the glomerulus?
    a. Renal artery, peritubular, arcuate, lobular, lobar, segmental, efferent arteriole
    b. Renal artery, arcuate, segmental, lobar, lobular, cortical radiate, afferent arteriole
    c. Renal artery, lobar, interlobar, lobular, cortical radiate, arcuate, efferent arteriole
    d. Renal artery, segmental, lobar, interlobar, arcuate, cortical radiate, afferent arteriole

16. Blood leaves the kidney's hilum via the:
    a. renal artery.
    b. inferior vena cava.
    c. efferent arteriole.
    d. renal vein.

17. As blood travels through the vessels that surround the nephrons, it exits the kidneys through a series of vessels that are in direct reverse of the arteries with one exception; there are
    a. no arcuate veins.
    b. no segmental veins.
    c. lobular or lobar veins.
    d. extra veins called the juxtaglomedullary veins.

18. In plasma, potassium is _____ than in glomerular filtrate.
    a. at the same concentration
    b. at a higher concentration
    c. at a lower concentration
    d. none of the above

19. What happens at the Bowman's capsule?
    a. Excretion
    b. Secretion
    c. Filtration
    d. Reabsorption

20. Angiotensinogen is secreted by the
    a. kidney.
    b. lungs.
    c. liver.
    d. adrenal cortex.

21. Which of the following is secreted at the nephron?
    a. Red blood cells and proteins
    b. White blood cells and sodium
    c. Water and glucose
    d. Ammonia and hydrogen ions

22. Glomerular filtrate flows from the renal corpuscle into the:
    a. loop of Henle.
    b. proximal convoluted tubules.
    c. distal convoluted tubules.
    d. collecting ducts.

23. Which of the following is either completely or partially reabsorbed, respectively, at the nephron?
    a. Red blood cells and potassium
    b. White blood cells and proteins
    c. Glucose and water
    d. Ammonia and hydrogen ions

24. Atrial natriuretic hormone (ANH) is released by the atria when blood volume
    a. increases.
    b. decreases.
    c. changes suddenly.
    d. there is no relationship between blood volume and ANH secretion.

25. When systemic blood pressure has decreased, what protective measures do the kidneys take?
    a. Vasoconstrict
    b. Vasodilate
    c. Shut down one kidney
    d. Nephrotic necrosis (spontaneous death of the nephrons)

MATCHING EXERCISES

Match each term with the appropriate definition.

Set 1

_____ 1. PKD
_____ 2. analgesic nephropathy
_____ 3. diabetes insipidus
_____ 4. diabetes mellitus
_____ 5. water toxicity
_____ 6. glomerulosclerosis
_____ 7. hemolytic uremic syndrome
_____ 8. kidney stones
_____ 9. hematuria
_____ 10. urinary tract infection

a. dangerously low blood sodium
b. nephrons are replaced by cysts
c. means blood in the urine
d. movement of fecal matter into urethra and bladder
e. scarring of portions of the renal corpuscles
f. may be caused by overuse of ibuprofen
g. insulin deficiency and hyperglycemia
h. RBC debris may block vessels to kidney
i. too little antidiuretic hormone being produce and secreted
j. can block kidney tubules

Set 2

_____ 1. rugae
_____ 2. diffusion
_____ 3. osmosis
_____ 4. voiding
_____ 5. filtration
_____ 6. secretion
_____ 7. reabsorption
_____ 8. autoregulation
_____ 9. vasoconstriction
_____ 10. vasodilation

a. increase of blood vessel diameter
b. decrease of blood vessel diameter
c. movement of ions and solutes from high to low concentration
d. urination
e. permit expansion of the urinary bladder
f. movement of substances from tubules to capillaries
g. controls blood pressure to nephrons
h. movement of water from low ion to high ion concentration
i.
j. movement of blood substances from glomerulus into capsule
k. movement of substances from capillaries to tubules

Set 3

_____ 1. ureter
_____ 2. urethra
_____ 3. kidney
_____ 4. bladder
_____ 5. nephron
_____ 6. renal hilum
_____ 7. renal pyramid
_____ 8. minor calyces
_____ 9. juxtaglomerular cells
_____ 10. peritubular capillaries

a. bean-shaped structure that filters blood and forms urine
b. functional unit of the kidney
c. striped areas in the renal medulla; collection of renal tubules
d. transport(s) urine from kidneys to bladder
e. transport(s) urine to outside the body
f. wrap(s) around nephrons; participate(s) in secretion and reabsorption
g. indentation on medial side of kidneys
h. monitor(s) blood flow to kidneys; secrete renin
i. receive(s) filtrate from collecting duct
j. hollow(s) holding structure for urine

Set 4

_____ 1. ADH
_____ 2. ANH
_____ 3. renin
_____ 4. angiotensin II
_____ 5. ACE
_____ 6. ACE inhibitor
_____ 7. epinephrine
_____ 8. aldosterone
_____ 9. juxtaglomerular cells
_____ 10. blood pressure

a. raise(s) blood pressure, secreted by kidney
b. lower(s) blood pressure
c. decrease(s) urination, increases sodium reabsorption
d. increases thirst and increases secretion of regulatory hormones
e. has(have) extensive feedback loop with kidney(s)
f. decrease(s) urination, secreted by hypothalamus
g. decrease(s) glomerular filtration by causing vasoconstriction of afferent arterioles
h. secrete(s) renin
i. convert(s) angiotensin I to angiotensin II in lungs
j. increase(s) urination, secreted by heart

FILL IN THE BLANK

Fill in the blanks to complete the following statements.

1. The three processes necessary to clean blood and make urine are _____, _____, and _____.

2. The vessels called _____ bring blood to the glomerulus, and the vessels called _____ leave the glomerulus with the unfiltered blood components.

3. The nephron is divided into two distinct parts called the _____ and the _____.

4. Beverages that contain _____ inhibit ADH secretion.

5. The noninvasive treatment to break up kidney stones, called _____, involves shock waves.

6. The leading cause of kidney failure in the United States is _____.

7. The hormone that acts to retain more sodium in the body is _____.

8. High blood pressure and urine glucose (sugar) are characteristic of a disorder called _____.

9. The three structures found at the renal hilum are the _____, _____, and _____.

10. The innermost region or layer of the kidney is the _____.

11. The functional unit of the kidney is the _____.

12. Glomerular filtrate flows from the proximal convoluted tubules into the _____.

13. When molecules move from the capillary network into the distal convoluted tubules, that movement is termed _____.

14. _____ converts angiotensinogen to angiotensin I.

15. Contraction of the urinary bladder muscles is controlled by _____ neurons of the autonomic nervous system.

16. The fibrous layer of connective tissue that covers the kidney is called the _____.

17. This substance, a waste product from muscle metabolism is one indicator of kidney function _____.

18. Hematuria is the presence of _____ in the urine.

19. The _____ in the brain gives humans voluntary control of urination.

20. _____ is the most common genetic cause of kidney disease.

21. One very important interaction, involved in blood pH, is the relationship of hydrogen ions (H⁺) and _____.

22. Infection with *E. coli* from eating undercooked meat can cause this disorder: _____.

23. The most obvious urinary symptom of untreated diabetes mellitus is _____.

24. If blood pH drops, more _____ will be secreted by the kidney.

25. If too little blood flows to the kidney, tissue damage called _____ will result and may eventually lead to kidney failure.

SHORT ANSWER

1. Why are urinary tract infections more common in women than in men?

2. In maintaining homeostasis and in reference to the urinary system, how does autoregulation work?

3. How does the body regulate pH if too much acid is present in the blood?

4. In what way are aldosterone and atrial natriuretic hormones antagonists?

5. Why would a person who survives a trauma resulting in massive blood loss fall victim to kidney damage or permanent renal failure?

___

___

___

___

LEARNING ACTIVITIES

1. Trace the flow of blood from the aorta through the kidney and back to the inferior vena cava. Can you do it?
2. Put together a group of students. Have each student write a scenario in which kidney function would be affected. Try to predict what would happen to urine output and blood pressure.
3. Nonsteroidal anti-inflammatory drugs (NSAIDs) are associated with renal failure in some individuals. Which ones? What makes NSAIDs apparently safe for some patients but not others? Use the internet to research the question.
4. Kidney disease and heart disease are often found in the same patients. Why? With a group of students, brainstorm the reasons why cardiovascular abnormalities are often found in kidney patients. Use the internet to check your hypotheses.

LABELING ACTIVITY

Label the parts of the kidney using Figure 16–2 as your guide.

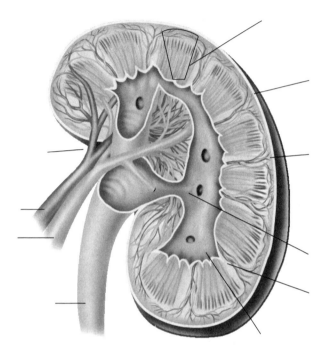

CROSSWORD PUZZLE

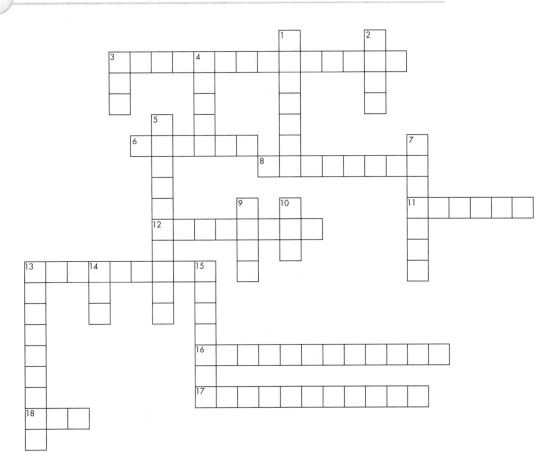

Across

3. protects glomerulus from typical blood pressure changes
6. organ that controls fluid and ion balance
8. tubule where most reabsorption and secretion takes place
11. outer layer of kidney, where filters are
12. arteriole leading to glomerulus
13. movement of substances from capillaries into tubule
16. movement of substances into bloodstream from tubules
17. where countercurrent circulation takes place (2 words)
18. made in hypothalamus, decreases urine production; abbreviation

Down

1. urinary _____ stores urine
2. part of brain which controls urination
3. enzyme which regulates blood pressure, abbreviation
4. secreted by kidney when blood flow decreases
5. movement of substances into kidney from blood at glomerulus
7. presence in urine is indicator of diabetes
9. nitrogen containing waste molecule
10. hormone which increases urine output; abbreviation
13. missing kidney vein
14. cannot normally pass through filter, abbreviation
15. fundamental functional unit of kidney

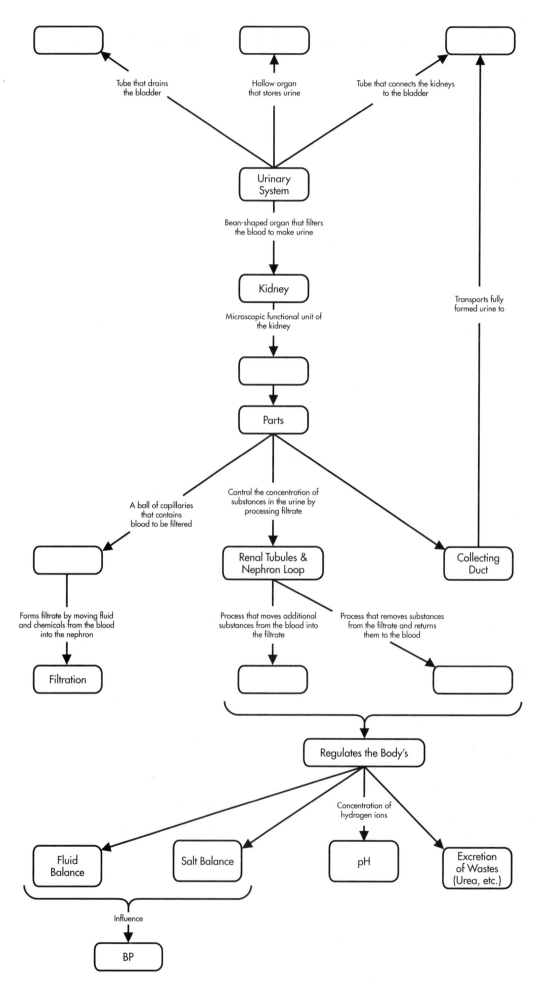

THE REPRODUCTIVE SYSTEM: REPLACEMENT AND REPAIR

MEDICAL TERMINOLOGY REVIEW

Define the following terms.
1. Endometriosis: _____
2. Amenorrhea: _____
3. Ectopic pregnancy: _____
4. Cryptorchidism: _____
5. Erectile dysfunction disorder: _____
6. Benign prostatic hyperplasia: _____
7. Hydrocele: _____
8. Androgen insensitivity: _____
9. Prostate cancer: _____
10. Premenstrual syndrome: _____

MULTIPLE CHOICE

Circle the letter of the correct answer.

1. The external opening of the vagina may be covered by a perforated membrane called the:
   a. prepuce.
   b. foreskin.
   c. hymen.
   d. fimbria.

2. BPH is a pathology marked by:
   a. breast polyps commonly seen in women over age 50.
   b. biological pelvic heliobacterium that affects prepubescent girls.
   c. prostate enlargement commonly seen in males over age 50.
   d. hermaphroditic pelvic organs caused by fetal hormone imbalance.

3. In patients with erectile dysfunction disorder:
   a. the penis lacks blood vessels in the shafts.
   b. the penis in unable to lose an erection.
   c. men are unable to make viable sperm.
   d. the penis is not able to have a full erection.

4. Uterine tubes are *not* the:
   a. birth canals.
   b. oviducts.
   c. fallopian tubes.
   d. site of fertilization.

5. How many chromosomes does a zygote have in each cell?
   a. 42
   b. 46
   c. 21
   d. 16 pairs

6. The primary male genitalia is/are the:
   a. penis.
   b. testicles.
   c. sperm.
   d. vas deferens.

7. Which of the following are parts of the spermatic cord?
   a. Vas deferens, ejaculatory duct, epididymis
   b. Testes, vas deferens, nerves
   c. Vas deferens, nerves, blood vessels
   d. Blood vessels, ejaculatory duct, penis

8. In most cases, vaginitis is caused by:
   a. microorganisms.
   b. macrooganisms.
   c. radiation.
   d. trauma.

9. In a pap test, scrapings from what area are examined for precancerous cells?
   a. Cervix
   b. Vaginal walls
   c. Uterine walls
   d. Ovarian surface

10. A hydrocele is an abnormal collection of fluid in the:
    a. ovaries.
    b. breasts.
    c. testes.
    d. uterus.

11. What may cause amenorrhea?
    a. Emotional distress
    b. Extreme dieting
    c. Poor health
    d. All of the above

12. When a vasectomy is performed, what is prevented from traveling out of the penis during intercourse?
    a. Semen
    b. Testosterone
    c. Sperm
    d. Urine

13. An IUD is a(n):
    a. inflammatory urethral disease.
    b. means of contraception.
    c. means of conception.
    d. gamete deformity.

14. When the loose skin covering the tip of the penis is removed, whether in infancy or adulthood, the male is then referred to as being:
    a. circumcised.
    b. impotent.
    c. aroused.
    d. neutered.

15. At what point is the developing human referred to as a fetus?
    a. At fertilization
    b. The eight-cell stage after fertilization
    c. At implantation
    d. Eight weeks after fertilization until birth

16. The time between the end of menses and ovulation is called the:
    a. luteal phase.
    b. follicular phase.
    c. secretory phase.
    d. interphase.

17. The fetus floats in a fluid called:
    a. amniotic.
    b. vestibular.
    c. semen.
    d. embryonic.

18. This hormone is secreted during the luteal phase to maintain the endometrium.
    a. Estrogen
    b. FSH
    c. LH
    d. Progesterone

19. Where is the prostate gland located?
    a. In the glans penis
    b. In the scrotum
    c. Inferior to the urinary bladder
    d. Lateral to the cervix

20. Which of the following layers of the uterus sheds when a woman has her period?
    a. Myometrium
    b. Perimetrium
    c. Functional layer of the mucosa
    d. Basal layer of the endometrium

21. The process of sorting chromosomes so that each gamete (egg or sperm) gets the right number of copies of the genetic material is called:
    a. meiosis.
    b. fertilization.
    c. reduction division.
    d. mitosis.

22. A surgeon wants to treat a tumor in the myometrium by occluding the arteries that serve that layer, without affecting the endometrium, perimetrium, or other pelvic structures. She will then attempt to occlude which arteries?
    a. Arcuate arteries
    b. Common iliac arteries
    c. Straight radial arteries
    d. Spiral radial arteries

23. Which structure of the female anatomy has great similarity to the penis in that it becomes engorged with blood during sexual arousal?
    a. Breast
    b. Ovaries
    c. Mons pubis
    d. Clitoris

24. What kind of feedback on the hypothalamus does testosterone exert?
    a. Negative
    b. Positive
    c. It changes during the cycle
    d. It is different in different people

25. Where do sperm mature?
    a. Epididymis
    b. Prostate
    c. Sertoli
    d. Penile shaft

MATCHING EXERCISES

Match each term with the appropriate definition.

Set 1

_____ 1. cryptorchidism
_____ 2. mastectomy
_____ 3. vasectomy
_____ 4. mastitis
_____ 5. ectopic pregnancy
_____ 6. abruptio placentae
_____ 7. perineum
_____ 8. breech
_____ 9. dysmenorrhea
_____ 10. follicle

a. the placenta tears away from the uterine walls
b. fertilized egg implants in fallopian tubes
c. egg and associated helper cells
d. when the testes do not descend during late fetal development
e. severing or tying off the vas deferens; a form of birth control
f. inflammation of the breast tissue
g. area between the vagina and anus
h. fetus coming through the birth canal buttocks first
i. difficult menstruation
j. removal of breast usually because of cancer or debilitating tumors

Set 2

_____ 1. gonads
_____ 2. areola
_____ 3. granulosa
_____ 4. vestibule
_____ 5. fimbria
_____ 6. corpus albicans
_____ 7. sertoli
_____ 8. tunica vaginalis
_____ 9. inguinal
_____ 10. tunica albuginea

a. space between labia minora where the urethra and vagina empty
b. most superficial layer of connective tissue surrounding testes
c. general term for both the ovaries and testes
d. fibrous capsule covering the ovaries
e. canal where the vas deferens passes from scrotum to trunk
f. helper cells for the sperm
g. nipple
h. helper cells surrounding the primary oocyte
i. ciliated projection on the distal portion of both uterine tubes
j. a degenerating structure in the ovaries

Set 3

_____ 1. semen
_____ 2. prolactin
_____ 3. oxytocin
_____ 4. testosterone
_____ 5. progesterone
_____ 6. estrogen
_____ 7. gonadotropin-releasing
_____ 8. follicle-stimulating hormone
_____ 9. luteinizing hormone
_____ 10. human chorionic

a. rising levels stimulate proliferation of the uterine lining
b. rising levels maintain the buildup of the endometrium
c. hormone responsible for maintaining the corpus luteum
d. substance containing sperm, mucus, sugars, and certain chemicals
e. hormone-regulating contraction of uterus and ejection of milk
f. responsible for masculinization at puberty
g. regulates production and secretion of hormone certain pituitary hormones
h. initiates the development of primary follicle
i. in females, a surge in this hormone is coupled with ovulation
j. hormone regulating the production of gonadotropin milk

Set 4

_____ 1. fallopian tube
_____ 2. vagina
_____ 3. ovaries
_____ 4. uterus
_____ 5. prostate
_____ 6. spermatic cord
_____ 7. epididymus
_____ 8. testes
_____ 9. seminiferous tubules
_____ 10. scrotum

a. female primary genitalia
b. secretes alkaline substance into semen
c. male primary genitalia
d. where fertilization takes place
e. houses testes
f. where sperm develop
g. transports sperm into abdominal cavity
h. birth canal
i. nourishes developing embryo
j. where sperm mature

FILL IN THE BLANK

Fill in the blanks to complete the following statements.

1. The typical genetic makeup of humans is that females have the sex chromosomes _____ and males have _____.

2. The urethra in males transports both _____ and _____.

3. The production of sperm is termed _____.

4. A(n) _____ refers to the expansion of the penis upon sexual arousal.

5. Milk-secreting sacs in the mammary lobules are called _____.

6. Between the two halves of the labia majora is an opening known as the _____ cleft.

7. The secretory phase of menstruation is also known as the _____ phase.

8. Sperm, in one of the many ducts, pass by the _____ just before flowing into the ejaculatory duct.

9. The type of cells that make up the human body are called _____ cells.

10. In males, luteinizing and follicle-stimulating hormones are produced and secreted by the _____.

11. If not surgically removed, the loose tissue called _____ normally covers the tip of the penis.

12. The isthmus of the uterine tubes are connected to the _____ of the uterus.

13. The primary male genitalia is/are the _____.

14. In humans, testosterone is first secreted _____.

15. The valvelike structure of the uterus called the _____ protrudes into the vagina, and its characteristic dilation marks a certain stage in delivery.

16. Cervical cancer can often be detected by a screening test known as a _____.

17. In an ectopic pregnancy the embryo implants in the _____.

18. Once it has been fertilized, an egg has _____ chromosomes and is called a(n) _____.

19. In men over age 50 with symptoms of urinary frequency and an enlarged prostate it is important to distinguish between _____ and _____.

20. The developing fetus is nurtured by the _____ via the umbilical cord.
21. Male sterilization is accomplished by a _____ for birth control purposes.
22. After ovulation, estrogen has a _____ feedback relationship with the pituitary.
23. The hormone _____ stimulates ovulation.
24. If a pregnancy results, _____ will be secreted.
25. _____ causes a change in the relationship between estrogen and LH and FSH.

SHORT ANSWER

1. Contrast the terms *menopause* and *menarche*.

2. Describe the three stages of labor.

3. Contrast the effects of estrogen and progesterone on the endometrium.

4. What determines the sex of a baby?

5. Trace the events of ejaculation from the scrotal sac to the release of semen into the vagina.

_____
_____
_____
_____

LEARNING ACTIVITIES

1. List as many similarities and differences as you can between the physiology of the male and female reproductive systems.
2. Without using your book, trace the path of a sperm from testes through ejaculation.
3. Hormonal abnormalities often lead to infertility in women. Speculate about the effects if a woman were missing one of the reproductive hormones. Use the internet to check your answer.
4. Use the internet to find out how the typical birth control pill works. Does it make sense given what you know about female hormones?
5. You have been given the task of developing a male contraceptive pill. What hormone would you block? What would be the potential side effects?

LABELING ACTIVITY

Label the parts of the male and female reproductive system and identify the organs described in the Function Boxes using Figure 5–17 in your textbook as a guide.

Organ	Primary Functions (female)
	Produce ova (eggs) and hormones
	Deliver ova or embryo to uterus; normal site of fertilization
	Site of development of offspring
	Site of sperm deposition; birth canal at delivery; provides passage of fluids during menstruation
	Erectile organ, produces pleasurable sensations during sexual act
	Contain glands that lubricate entrance to vagina
	Produce milk that nourishes newborn infant

Organ	Primary Functions (male)
	Produce sperm and hormones
	Site of sperm maturation
	Conducts sperm between epididymis and prostate
	Secrete fluid that makes up much of the volume of semen
	Secretes buffers and fluid
	Conducts semen to exterior
	Erectile organ used to deposit sperm in the vagina of a female; produces pleasurable sensations during sexual act
	Surrounds and positions the testes

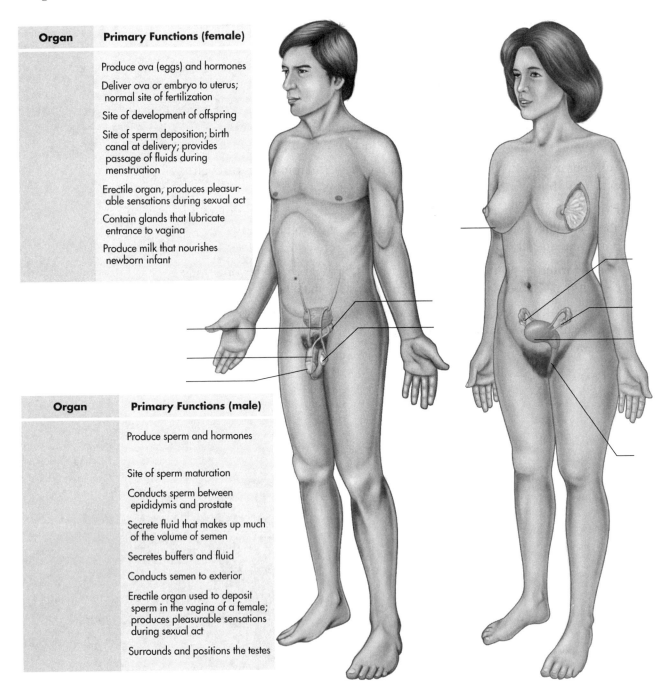

CROSSWORD PUZZLE

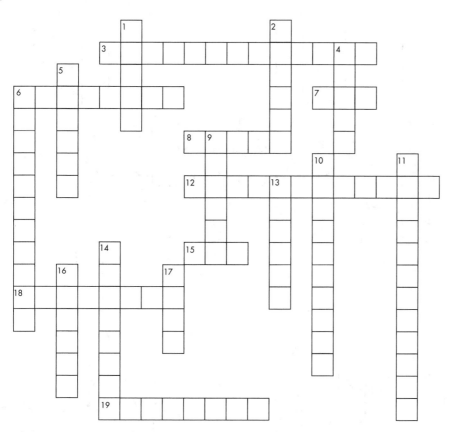

Across

3. union of sperm and egg
6. stiffening of penis
7. _____ test, test for cervical cancer
8. female external genitalia
12. movement of fluid and tissue down the vagina
15. stimulates maturation of gametes
18. stimulate uterine contractions
19. controls development of female secondary sexual characters

Down

1. sperm delivery organ
2. birth canal
4. female primary genitalia
5. time during which a woman is menstruating
6. ejection of sperm from penis
9. where fertilized egg implants
10. layer of endometrium that is shed each month
11. secretes progesterone after ovulation
13. male primary genitalia
14. can be enlarged in older men
16. fertilized egg
17. stimulates secretion of FSH and LH

Name _____

CONCEPT MAP

Fill in the empty boxes with an appropriate term. Use the clues provided.

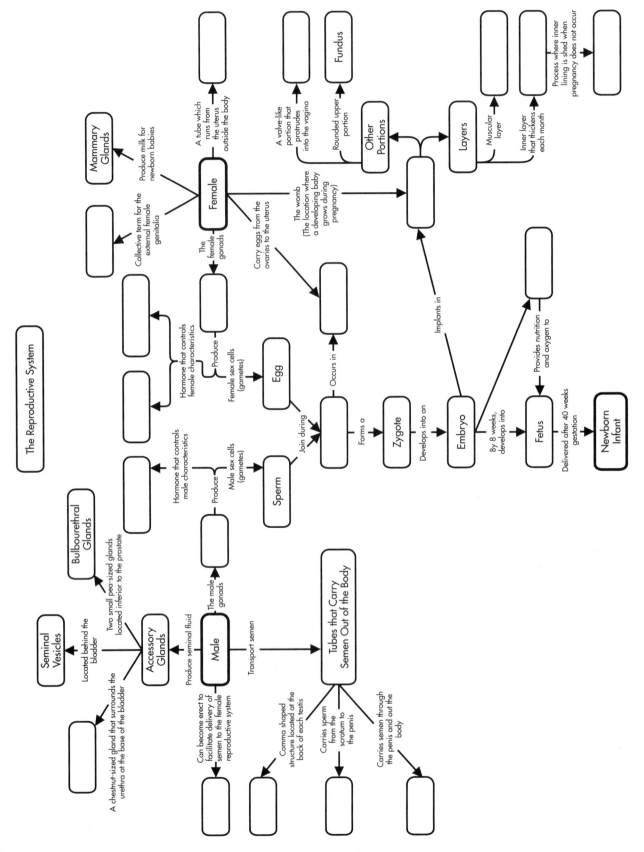

THE JOURNEY'S END: NOW WHAT?

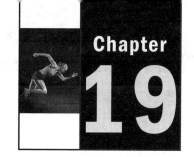

Chapter 19

MEDICAL TERMINOLGY REVIEW

Define the following terms.
1. DNA fingerprinting: _____
2. Geriatric: _____
3. Polypharmacy: _____
4. Chemotherapy: _____
5. Radiation: _____
6. Immunotherapy: _____
7. Sexually transmitted infection: _____
8. Melanoma: _____
9. Colonoscopy: _____
10. Drug compliance: _____

MULTIPLE CHOICE

Circle the letter of the correct answer.

1. Bone scouring is an indication of:
   a. tuberculosis.
   b. hepatitis.
   c. calcium deficiency.
   d. high-impact mechanical stress.

2. Which nerve is damaged in carpal tunnel syndrome?
   a. Median
   b. Acoustic
   c. Sciatic
   d. Radial

3. What bone fragment, showing evidence of primitive surgery, was found in a 400-year-old trash dump?
   a. Skull
   b. Femur
   c. Rib
   d. Sacrum

4. Who was Josef Mengele?
   a. The Merciless Hooded Ghost responsible for the brutality against Native Americans between 1812 and 1831
   b. The Fearless Ace responsible for "downing" several Allied fighter jets
   c. The Consignor of the Hanoi Hilton responsible for the torture of many prisoners of war during the Vietnam War
   d. The Angel of Death responsible for the deaths of many people during World War II

5. According to your text, what substance containing thallium was intentionally and secretly fed to a victim, causing his death?
   a. Rat poison
   b. Drain cleaner
   c. Paint thinner
   d. Motor oil

6. Which of the following is true about fingerprints?
   a. Only identical twins have the same fingerprints.
   b. They are friction ridges on the hands and feet.
   c. They are only fully formed between the first and second year of life.
   d. All of the above

7. DNA fingerprinting helped determine that Thomas Jefferson, the third president of the United States, or a relative:
   a. Murdered his first wife
   b. Burglarized the White House repeatedly
   c. Fathered children of his slave
   d. Had Alzheimer's disease

8. In older adults, what changes are seen in the taste buds?
   a. The acuity of salt receptors becomes more sensitive
   b. The number of taste buds increases
   c. Sweet tastes become less discernable than bitter tastes
   d. All of the above

9. Although bone loss occurs in both men and women, the highest percentage bone loss in women can be seen:
   a. ten years after menopause.
   b. in the first five years postmenopause.
   c. six months prior to menopause.
   d. after age 70.

10. As humans age:
    a. heart valves become soft.
    b. cardiac output decreases.
    c. blood pressure decreases.
    d. All of the above

11. Which of the following is true of the female pelvis?
    a. The female pelvis is more funnel-shaped than the male pelvis.
    b. The female pelvis has a pubic angle of 90 degrees.
    c. The female pelvis is stronger than the male pelvis.
    d. The female pelvis is lighter than the male pelvis.

12. In forensic science, which anatomical structure is examined for evidence of tuberculosis?
    a. The skin
    b. The nasal apertures
    c. The retina of the left eye
    d. The ends of long bones

13. In older adults, changes in the integumentary system include:
    a. increased skin delicacy.
    b. loss of elasticity.
    c. multiple lesions.
    d. All of the above

14. Stress:
    a. is not a natural part of life and must be controlled.
    b. gives a false sense of security and protection.
    c. is good and necessary, but chronic stress may be problematic.
    d. All of the above

15. What is recommended for maintaining healthy bones?
    a. Calcium and vitamins
    b. Weight-bearing exercises
    c. Repetitive motion such as typing
    d. a and b

16. What may cause carpal tunnel syndrome?
    a. Bright lights and abuse of such drugs as ecstasy
    b. Weight-bearing exercises
    c. Loud sounds and high pitches
    d. Repetitive motion such as playing the piano

17. For optimum health, how many times per week should a person exercise?
    a. 1-3 days
    b. 3-5 days
    c. 3-7 days
    d. As time permits
18. What technique was initially used to confirm that Wolfgang Gerhard was really Josef Mengele?
    a. Video skull–face superimposition
    b. Fingerprints
    c. Voice recognition
    d. Reverse psychology and multiple interviews
19. Which of the following has/have an adverse effect on the cardiovascular system?
    a. Alcohol
    b. Smoking
    c. Saturated fats
    d. All of the above
20. Why can high doses of vitamin A, D, E, and K actually harm the body?
    a. Being water soluble, they tax the kidneys
    b. They deteriorate the stomach's lining
    c. They can build up to a toxic level
    d. They prevent absorption of proteins and carbohydrates
21. What is needed in order to identify a criminal suspect through DNA fingerprinting?
    a. Both blood and reproductive fluid from a crime scene
    b. Both DNA from a crime scene and a known DNA sample from the accused
    c. Both DNA from the mother and father of the accused
    d. Only the DNA from the crime scene
22. The simplest and most effective way to stop the spread of infections is:
    a. avoid contact.
    b. wash hands.
    c. drink more water.
    d. take antibiotics.
23. What kind of agent is an antibiotic cream or tablet?
    a. Antifungal
    b. Antiviral
    c. Antiprotozoan
    d. Antibacterial
24. Which of the following is/are considered diuretics?
    a. Water
    b. Beer
    c. Grape juice
    d. a and c
25. The ability to roll your tongue is:
    a. gender-specific.
    b. learned.
    c. an inherited trait.
    d. race-specific.

MATCHING EXERCISES

Match each term with the appropriate definition.

Set 1

_____ 1. vitamin A
_____ 2. calcium
_____ 3. vitamin B_1
_____ 4. vitamin B_{12}
_____ 5. vitamin C
_____ 6. niacin
_____ 7. vitamin E
_____ 8. vitamin K
_____ 9. vitamin D
_____ 10. folic acid

a. aids in the absorption of calcium from the gut
b. facilitates fat synthesis and glycolysis
c. recommended for proper night vision
d. raw material for bones and teeth
e. needed for hemolytic resistance of RBCs
f. needed to prevent spina bifida
g. needed for carbohydrate metabolism and normal digestion and appetite
h. used to treat pernicious anemia
i. needed for proper blood clotting
j. aids in the absorption of iron

Set 2

_____ 1. SIDS
_____ 2. black lung
_____ 3. lead poisoning
_____ 4. genital warts
_____ 5. syphilis
_____ 6. herpes
_____ 7. gonorrhea
_____ 8. chlamydia
_____ 9. melanoma
_____ 10. tuberculosis

a. common among coalminers
b. human papilloma virus
c. presents with fluid-filled vesicles on the gentalia
d. presents with swollen testes and inflamed cervix
e. skin cancer
f. normally thought of as a bacterial pulmonary disease
g. associated with infants
h. from pewter plates
i. presents with degeneration of the nervous system
j. presents with purulent discharge and abnormal menstruation

Set 3

Match the following systems with their appropriate age-related and/or wellness concerns.

_____ 1. reproductive system
_____ 2. immune system
_____ 3. sensory system
_____ 4. endocrine system
_____ 5. brain and nervous system
_____ 6. respiratory system
_____ 7. skeletal system
_____ 8. integumentary system
_____ 9. cardiovascular system
_____ 10. urinary system

a. incontinence
b. pain and stress
c. clogged vessels
d. antibiotics abuse
e. smoking and emphysema
f. high level of noise
g. steroid abuse
h. skin cancer
i. carpal tunnel syndrome
j. smoking and SIDS

Set 4

_____ 1. mammography
_____ 2. colonoscopy
_____ 3. Pap test
_____ 4. forensic tests
_____ 5. skull-face superimposition
_____ 6. DNA fingerprinting
_____ 7. Snellen eye chart
_____ 8. sentinel lymph node mapping and biopsy
_____ 9. fingerprints
_____ 10. bone density

a. identification
b. cervical cancer
c. identification of fluids
d. visual acuity
e. osteoporosis
f. breast cancer
g. crime scene technique in use for a century
h. crime
i. colon cancer
j. cancer spread

FILL IN THE BLANK

Fill in the blanks to complete the following statements.

1. Ancient _____ were stricken with tuberculosis, as investigators discovered by examining their bones.
2. One expected change related to aging is that nails become _____ and skin becomes _____.
3. Administering many drugs at the same time is termed _____.
4. In the absence of disease, the brain continues to mature up to the age of _____.
5. Bone density usually reaches its greatest peak at _____.
6. In general, as an individual ages, he or she loses _____ and _____ and gains _____.
7. A pap test is used for determining cancer of the _____.
8. Anabolic steroids are closely related to the hormone _____.
9. A mammogram is a test for cancer of the _____.
10. Approximately _____ people die annually in the United States because of smoking-related disease.
11. The cancer treatment that uses energy waves rather than chemicals to shrink tumors is called _____ therapy.
12. Clients who have the procedure called _____ usually are 26 percent less likely to have their cancer return within 5 years than clients who only have the tumor removed.

13. Smoking can lead to chronic respiratory diseases such as _____, _____, and _____.
14. CIPA is the acronym for _____.
15. According to the text, thallium was found in a victim's _____, which linked the wife to the murder.
16. People older than age 85 are classified as _____ old.
17. Loss of appetite, grumpiness, and pallor may be signs of _____.
18. Decreased _____ function may lead to overmedication in older patients.
19. The _____ population is the fastest-growing population in the United States.
20. Vitamin _____ is necessary for visual health.
21. Antibiotic _____ results from improper use of antibiotics.
22. Research appears to indicate that vitamins and minerals from _____ are better utilized than are synthetic pills.
23. Poor oral hygiene increases the risk of _____.
24. The hallmark sign of aging is the decreased ability to maintain _____.
25. Genes, radiation, sunlight exposure, smoking, fatty foods, viruses, and chemical exposure can all trigger _____.

SHORT ANSWER

1. How does the sexually transmitted infection HPV present itself in both males and females?

   _____
   _____
   _____
   _____

2. Besides completely staying out of the sun, in what ways can people prevent excessive sun exposure?

   _____
   _____
   _____
   _____

3. What are the serious side effects of steroid abuse in both men and women?

    _____
    _____
    _____
    _____

4. In what ways can untreated pain affect older adults?

    _____
    _____
    _____
    _____

5. Why, during the Middle Ages, were tomatoes believed to be poisonous?

    _____
    _____
    _____
    _____

LEARNING ACTIVITIES

1. Select a vitamin from the list in the book and brainstorm what kind of symptoms would result from a deficit of that vitamin. Use the internet to check your hypothesis.

2. Polypharmacy is a real problem for many older patients. Choose a combination of drugs that might be taken together—for example, cholesterol meds, calcium supplements, and blood pressure medication. Use the Internet to find out the potential interactions between the drugs. Start with two drugs, then go to three or even four. Does it get harder to predict the potential interactions as more drugs are added to the list? Why or why not?

3. Examine your lifestyle choices. How healthy are you? Do you engage in risky behavior? Do you get enough exercise? Eat right? How might your lifestyle choices today influence your health 40 years from now? Review the list of *Healthy People 2020* Topics and Objectives on the HealthyPeople.gov website. How many of these objectives do you currently meet? What objectives *should* you work on? Why?

4. Some environmental factors are known to increase the risk of developing certain cancers. List the ones you can off the top of your head and from the textbook. Then do some research. Which cancers are influenced by environmental factors? Which factors?

5. Bacteria have increasingly become resistant to antibiotics. What factors contribute to antibiotics resistance?

CROSSWORD PUZZLE

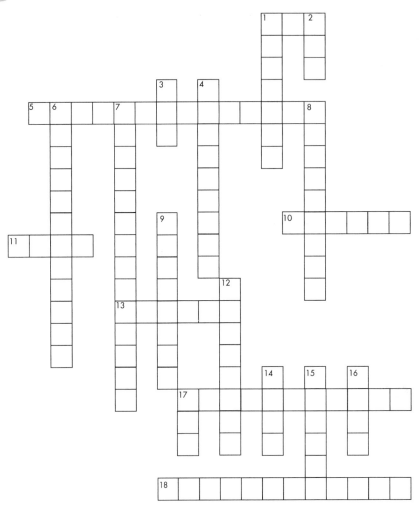

Across
1. abbreviation, sexually transmitted disease
5. comparing one DNA sample to another is DNA _____
10. a little is healthy, but chronic is bad
11. can be a timeline of chemical exposure
13. the uncontrolled reproductionn and spread of abnormal cells
17. birth defect that can be prevented by vitamin B supplements (2 words)
18. taking many drugs at the same time

Down
1. millions of lives could be saved if people quit _____
2. the genetic material is in this molecule
3. virus that causes many cases of cervical cancer (abbreviation)
4. _____ choices have profound health effects
6. many older people suffer this uninary system disorder
7. many cancer deaths can be prevented by _____ (2 words)
8. referring to the elderly
9. _____ science is the application of science to crime
12. fingerprints are _____ ridges
14. many older patients are undermedicated for _____
15. this taste increases in intensity with age
16. becoming healthy involves changes in _____ and exercise
17. the _____ of the victim is often obvious from the pelvis

Name _____

CONCEPT MAP

Fill in the empty boxes with an appropriate term using the clues provided.

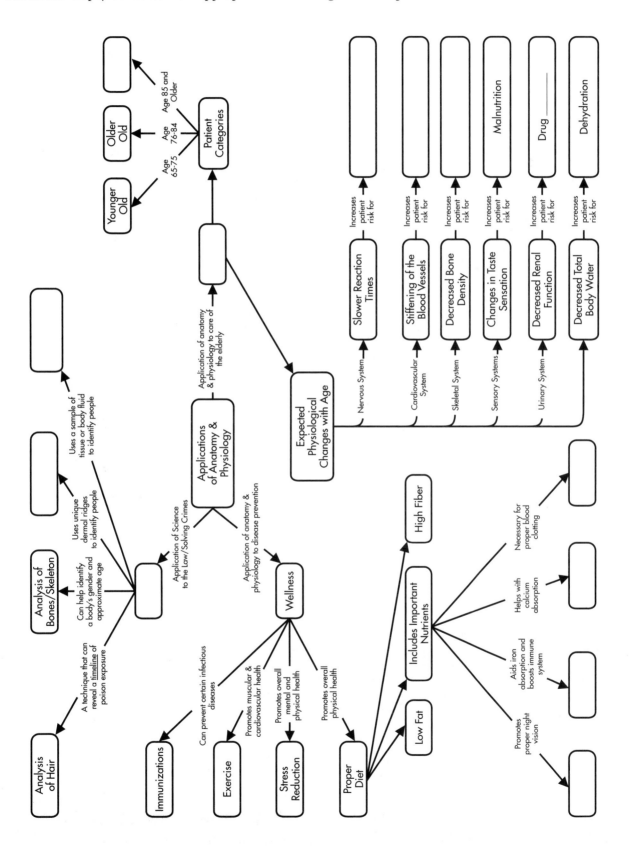

CHAPTER 1
ANSWER KEY

MEDICAL TERMINOLOGY REVIEW

1. Pathology: The study of disease
2. Physiology: The study of function
3. Etiology: Cause of a disease
4. Anatomy: The study of a structure
5. Diagnosis: Identification of disease based on signs and symptoms
6. Prognosis: Prediction of the outcome of a disease
7. Homeostasis: The ability of the body to maintain constant internal environment
8. Signs: Definitive, objective, measurable indicators of illness
9. Symptoms: Subjective measures of disease, perceived by the patient
10. Negative feedback: Opposes a change away from set point

MULTIPLE CHOICE

1. b
2. c
3. a
4. a
5. d
6. d
7. b
8. b
9. b
10. a
11. b
12. c
13. d
14. c
15. d
16. c
17. c
18. d
19. b
20. d
21. a
22. c
23. a
24. c
25. a

MATCHING EXERCISES

Set 1	Set 2	Set 3	Set 4
1. h	1. i	1. f	1. e
2. l	2. c	2. h	2. i
3. e	3. m	3. d	3. a
4. a	4. a	4. c	4. f
5. f	5. j	5. b	5. d
6. j	6. k	6. g	6. h
7. c	7. l	7. e	7. c
8. i	8. b	8. a	8. j
9. g	9. e	9. i	9. g
10. d	10. g	10. j	10. b

FILL IN THE BLANK

1. STAT
2. NPO
3. negative feedback
4. International System of Units/metric
5. nephrectomy
6. dermatology
7. hepatitis
8. cholecystectomy
9. homeostasis
10. etiology
11. diagnosis
12. prognosis
13. microscopic
14. syndrome
15. vital
16. kilograms (kg)
17. microscope
18. symptoms
19. etiology
20. diagnosis
21. treatment
22. prognosis
23. symptom
24. emia
25. positive

SHORT ANSWER

1. *Sign* and *symptom* are terms often used interchangeably but each has its own specific definition. A sign is a more objective indicator (pulse rate) of illness, and a symptom is a more subjective (pain behind the eyes, for example) indicator of illness.

2. Homeostasis is the body's ability to maintain a constant internal environment. Sensory receptors measure variables and compare them to a set point, the ideal value of the variable. A control center determines a course of action to maintain set point and effectors carry out the orders from the control center, either raising or lowering the variable to bring it back to set point.

3. *Anatomy* and *physiology* are the study of both the structure and function of the internal and external structure of plants, animals, or for the focus of this text, the human body.

4. The metric system is much easier to use because it is based on multiples of ten. The U.S. Customary System (USCS) requires remembering a number of unrelated measurements. Conversions between units are difficult.

5. Each medical term has a basic structure called the *word root*. It is combined with prefixes and suffixes that can change its meaning. Prefixes come before the word root, whereas suffixes come after the word root.

CROSSWORD PUZZLE

Across

2. metric system weight measurement
4. abbreviation for complete blood count
5. the study of function
8. word root meaning "bone"
12. suffix meaning "enlarged"
14. means "inflammation of"
18. feedback that resists a change

Down

1. the study of structure
3. prefix meaning "tissue"
4. word root for "cell"
5. feedback that enhances a change
6. subjective indicator of disease
7. means "condition of"
9. objective, measurable indicator of disease
10. within
11. prefix for "difficult"
13. cause of disease
15. ideal normal value
16. metric volume measurement
17. prefix meaning "around"

CONCEPT MAP

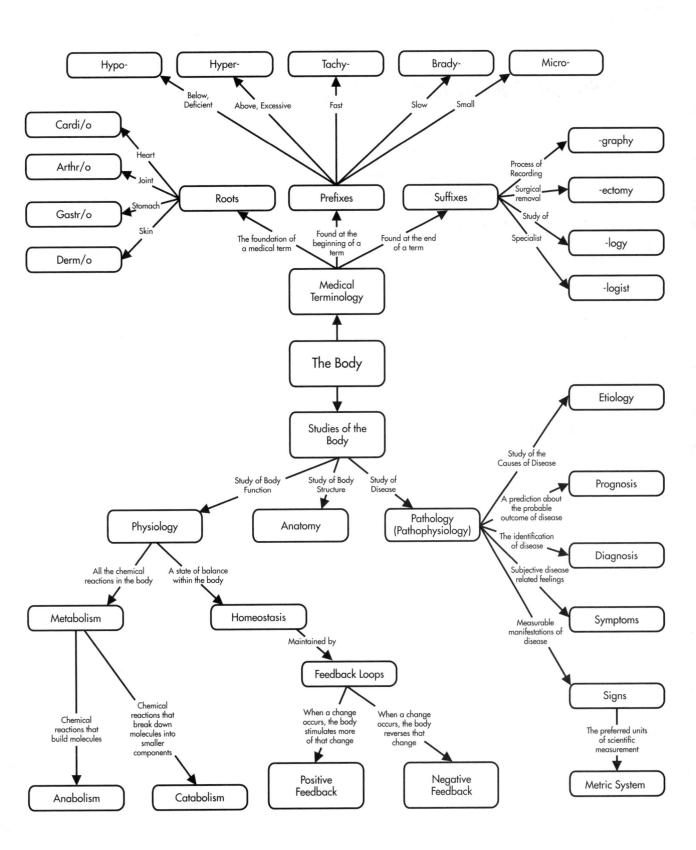

CHAPTER 2
ANSWER KEY

MEDICAL TERMINOLOGY REVIEW

1. Patellar: Pertaining to the knee cap
2. Plantar: Pertaining to the sole of foot
3. Antecubital: Pertaining to the area anterior to elbow
4. Femoral: Pertaining to the thigh
5. Axillary: Pertaining to the armpit
6. Carpal: Pertaining to the wrist
7. Cervical: Pertaining to the neck
8. Lumbar: Pertaining to the lower back
9. Umbilical: Pertaining to the navel
10. Thoracic: Pertaining to the chest

MULTIPLE CHOICE

1. b
2. b
3. a
4. c
5. a
6. d
7. d
8. c
9. a
10. a
11. b
12. d
13. a
14. d
15. b
16. d
17. d
18. c
19. a
20. a
21. c
22. d
23. a
24. c
25. d

Copyright © 2020 by Pearson Education, Inc.

MATCHING EXERCISES

Set 1	Set 2	Set 3	Set 4
1. h	1. e	1. f	1. j
2. j	2. l	2. d	2. e
3. g	3. h	3. b	3. g
4. a	4. a	4. c	4. b
5. i	5. g	5. g	5. h
6. e	6. c	6. j	6. a
7. f	7. j	7. a	7. i
8. l	8. i	8. i	8. c
9. c	9. b	9. e	9. f
10. b	10. f	10. k	10. k

FILL IN THE BLANK

1. dorsal
2. cheek
3. psoas
4. pleural
5. frontal/coronal
6. horizontal/transverse
7. pelvic
8. right lumbar
9. hypogastric
10. iliac
11. dorsal recumbent
12. epigastric
13. superior/proximal
14. medial
15. distal
16. patient's
17. lower back
18. Ultrasound
19. x-ray
20. MRI
21. Bone
22. occipital
23. patella
24. cheek
25. liver

SHORT ANSWER

1. The divisions of the abdominal regions include the right and left lower quadrants and the right and left upper quadrants.

2. The coronal/frontal plane divides the body into anterior and posterior sections. The sagittal plane divides the body into right and left sections (the median/midsagittal divides it in half). The transverse plan divides the body into superior and inferior sections.

3. The anatomical position is a human standing erect, face forward, with feet parallel and arms hanging at the side, with palms facing forward.

4. Proximal to the hips is the upper thigh or the femoral region. The leg or the crural region and the kneecap or the patella are inferior to the thigh on the anterior of the leg. The back of the knee or the popliteal region is posterior to the patella. The foot or the pedal region is the most distal part of the limb. The foot by itself includes the top, or the dorsum, and the sole, or the plantar surface.

5. The larger anterior cavity is subdivided into two main cavities called the thoracic cavity and abdominopelvic cavity. These cavities are physically separated by a large, dome-shaped muscle called the diaphragm, which is used for breathing. The thoracic cavity contains the heart, lungs, and large blood vessels. The heart has its own small cavity called the pericardial cavity. The abdominopelvic cavity contains the digestive organs, such as the stomach, intestines, liver, gallbladder, pancreas, and spleen in the superior or abdominal portion. The inferior portion, called the pelvic cavity, contains the urinary and reproductive organs and the last part of the large intestine. A posterior cavity is located in the back of the body and consists of the cranial cavity, which houses the brain, and the spinal cavity (vertebral cavity), which contains the spinal cord.

LABELING ACTIVITY

See Figure 2–8 in the textbook for comparison.

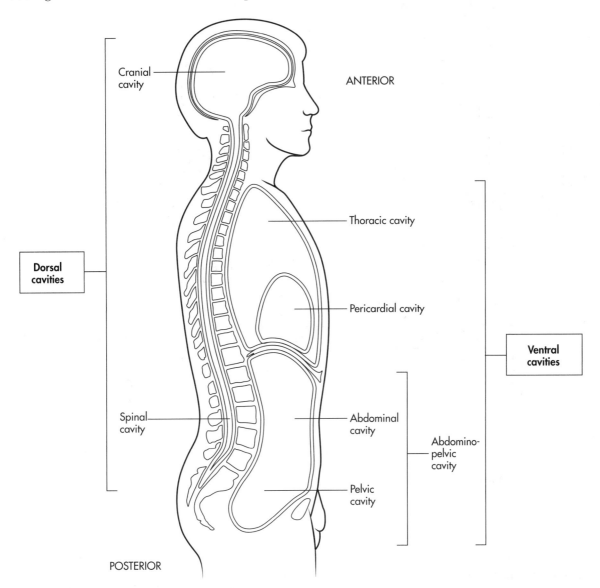

CROSSWORD PUZZLE

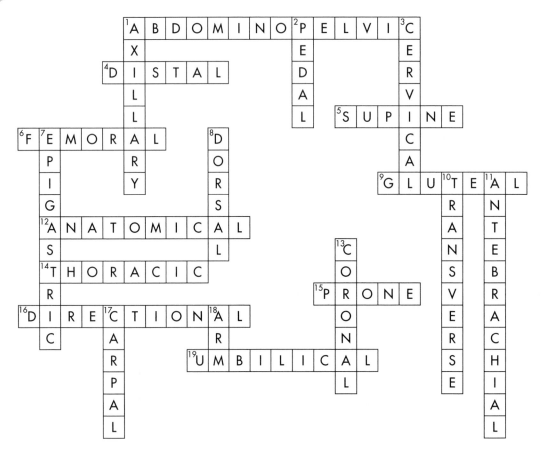

Across
1. body cavity inferior to the diaphragm
4. far from origin
5. face up
6. thigh
9. buttocks
12. standard body position
14. cavity superior to diaphragm
15. face down
16. _____ terms; used to describe anatomy
19. abdominal region surrounding belly button

Down
1. armpit
2. foot
3. neck
7. abdominal region on top of stomach
8. back
10. divides body into superior and inferior sections
11. forearm
13. divides body into anterior and posterior parts
17. wrist
18. brachial

CONCEPT MAP

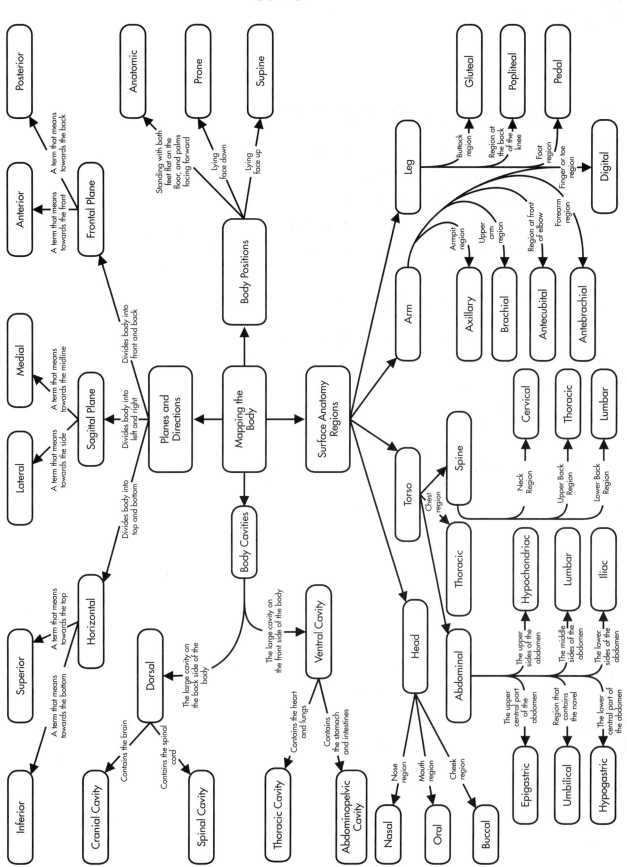

CHAPTER 3
ANSWER KEY

MEDICAL TERMINOLOGY REVIEW

1. Steroid: Ringed lipids, acts as powerful hormone
2. pH: Scale used to measure acidity, pH 7 is neutral
3. Electrolyte: Physiologically important ions
4. Hydrophobic: Molecules that cannot mix with water, nonpolar
5. Solution: A substance (the solute) dissolved in a liquid (solvent)
6. Concentration: The amount of solute in a solution
7. Biological molecules: Carbon-containing molecules found in living things
8. Glucose: A simple sugar necessary for cell metabolism
9. Glycogen: Molecule used for storing glucose
10. Metabolism: All the chemical reactions in the cell

MULTIPLE CHOICE

1. b
2. c
3. a
4. c
5. d
6. a
7. d
8. b
9. c
10. b
11. c
12. c
13. a
14. d
15. d
16. c
17. b
18. c
19. a
20. b
21. d
22. b
23. c
24. c
25. d

MATCHING EXERCISES

Set 1	Set 2	Set 3	Set 4
1. d	1. j	1. d	1. d
2. a	2. a	2. i	2. h
3. i	3. e	3. b	3. b
4. f	4. g	4. a	4. f
5. b	5. c	5. g	5. j
6. h	6. b	6. j	6. c
7. j	7. d	7. e	7. e
8. c	8. i	8. f	8. a
9. e	9. f	9. c	9. g
10. g	10. h	10. h	10. i

FILL IN THE BLANK

1. molecules
2. first two letters
3. saturated
4. protons
5. charged
6. electrolytes
7. urinary
8. bicarbonate
9. acid
10. polar covalent
11. solvent
12. build up
13. speed up
14. specific
15. mitochondria
16. carbon dioxide, water
17. ADP
18. acid
19. dehydration synthesis
20. electrons
21. peptide bond
22. diluent
23. element
24. protein
25. 7

SHORT ANSWER

1. Substrates bind to the enzyme. The enzyme brings the substrates close together so they can react faster, speeding up the reaction. The enzyme then releases the product and goes back for more substrates. Enzymes can carry only certain substrates (specificity).

2. Carbohydrates have two hydrogens and one oxygen for each carbon. They are generally used for energy storage and are hydrophilic. Proteins are long chains of amino acids held together by peptide bonds, so they have nitrogen in their backbone. They have many different functions. Lipids have mainly carbon and hydrogen with very little oxygen so they are hydrophobic. Lipids come in a variety of configurations and have many different functions. Nucleic acids, RNA and DNA, are long chains of nucleotides (phosphate, sugar, base). They are part of the genetic code.

3. Ionic bonds result when one atom donates electrons to the other. These molecules are charged. In covalent bonds, electrons are shared. However, unequal sharing results in a polar covalent bond. Molecules with polar covalent bonds carry a charge.

4. In cellular respiration, glucose is used to make ATP. Oxygen is also required. In the process, carbon dioxide and water are given off as waste products.

5. Metabolism consists of all the reactions that happen in a cell. The two subdivisions of metabolism are anabolism and catabolism. Anabolism is the building up of complex structures using simpler compounds, like amino acids being used to build protein. Catabolism is the tearing down of complex material into smaller material, like the breaking down of food into its nutritional components.

CROSSWORD PUZZLE

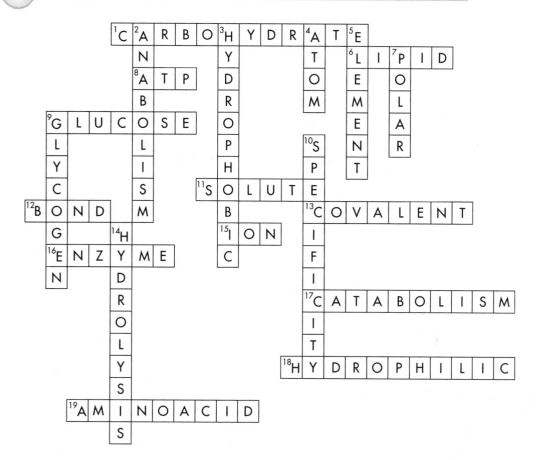

Across

1. has molecular formula CH₂O
6. has lots of H and C but little O
8. high energy molecule made during cellular respiration
9. monosaccharide, necessary for cellular respiration
11. dissolved in a solution
12. hydrogen _____ occurs between adjacent water molecules
13. when atoms share electrons
15. charged atom or molecule
16. speeds up rates of biological reactions
17. breaking down large molecules
18. water loving
19. the building block of protein (2 words)

Down

2. building large molecules out of small ones
3. will not mix with water
4. smallest recognizable unit of an element
5. smallest unit of specific type of matter
7. charged
9. polysaccharide
10. only certain molecules can fit in a binding site
14. adding water to split molecules

CONCEPT MAP

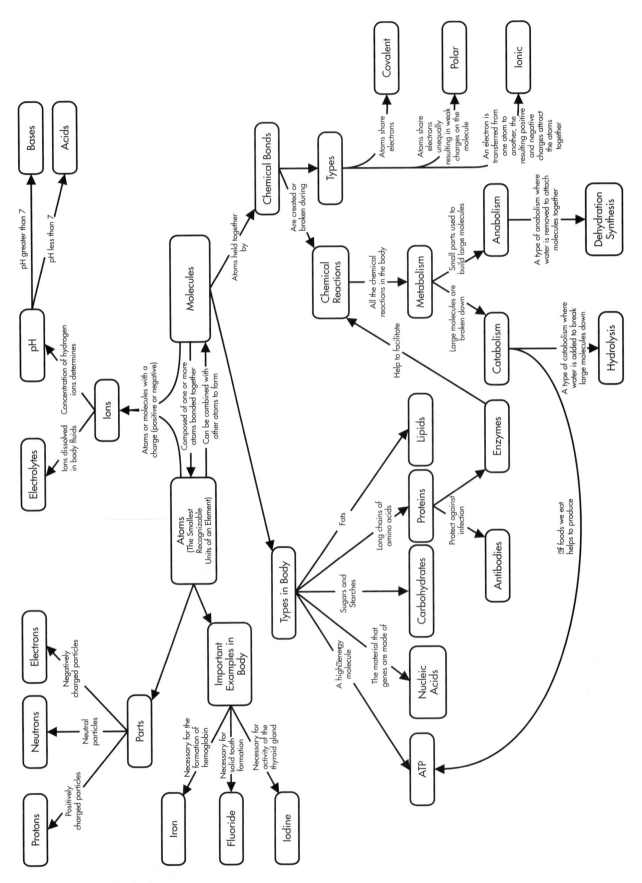

CHAPTER 4
ANSWER KEY

MEDICAL TERMINOLOGY REVIEW

1. Nucleus: Control center of cell, contains DNA
2. Cellular respiration: Series of cellular reactions that use glucose and oxygen to make ATP, a high-energy molecule
3. Cancer: Uncontrolled reproduction and spread of abnormal cells
4. Semipermeable: Some substances can pass through easily and some cannot
5. Antibiotic: Drug that kills bacteria without harming our cells
6. Mitosis: Cell division in eukaryotic cells
7. Organelle: Subcellular structures with specific jobs
8. Pathogen: An organism that harms another via infection
9. Virus: A pathogen without the ability to reproduce; hijacks host cell
10. Bacteria: A prokaryotic cell that may or may not be pathogenic

MULTIPLE CHOICE

1. b
2. d
3. d
4. c
5. a
6. a
7. c
8. b
9. d
10. c
11. b
12. c
13. a
14. b
15. b
16. c
17. a
18. a
19. a
20. b
21. a
22. c
23. a
24. c
25. b

MATCHING EXERCISES

Set 1	Set 2	Set 3	Set 4
1. g	1. i	1. a	1. d
2. d	2. b	2. f	2. f
3. c	3. h	3. i	3. h
4. a	4. d	4. e	4. b
5. i	5. c	5. d	5. e
6. f	6. a	6. b	6. j
7. b	7. j	7. j	7. a
8. j	8. g	8. c	8. c
9. h	9. e	9. h	9. g
10. e	10. f	10. g	10. i

FILL IN THE BLANK

1. diffusion
2. phagocytosis
3. adenosine triphosphate
4. active transport pumps
5. DNA
6. cilia
7. virus
8. vitamin K
9. spores
10. solute
11. phosphate
12. bacteria
13. cytokinesis
14. cell
15. malaria
16. pathogen
17. lysosomes
18. ATP
19. proteins
20. mitochondria
21. Cancer
22. oxygen
23. prophase
24. metastasis
25. Antibiotics

SHORT ANSWER

1. The cell membrane is responsible for allowing materials in and out of the cell.

2. Antibiotics are effective only against prokaryotic cells, so they kill bacteria but not the host cell or any virus, since viruses are not cells. Antiviral drugs can only target viruses by targeting the host cells, since viruses hijack cells.

3. Prophase (*pro* = before)—the nucleus disappears, the chromosomes become visible, and a set of chromosomal anchor lines or guide wires, the spindle, forms. Metaphase (*meta* = between)—the chromosomes line up in the center of the cells. Anaphase (*an* = without)—the chromosomes split, and the spindles pull them apart. Telophase (*telo* = the end)—the chromosomes go to the far end of the cell, the spindle disappears, and the nuclei reappear.

4. Passive transport requires no extra energy and includes such specific transports as diffusion, osmosis, and filtration. Active transport requires energy in the form of adenosine triphosphate and includes active pump, endocytosis, and exocytosis.

5. ATP is a high-energy molecule that has three phosphate groups. Each bond with phosphate stores energy, so when ATP loses a phosphate and becomes ADP (adensine diphosphate), it gives off energy that can be used to power cell metabolism.

LABELING ACTIVITY

See Figure 4–1 in the textbook for comparison.

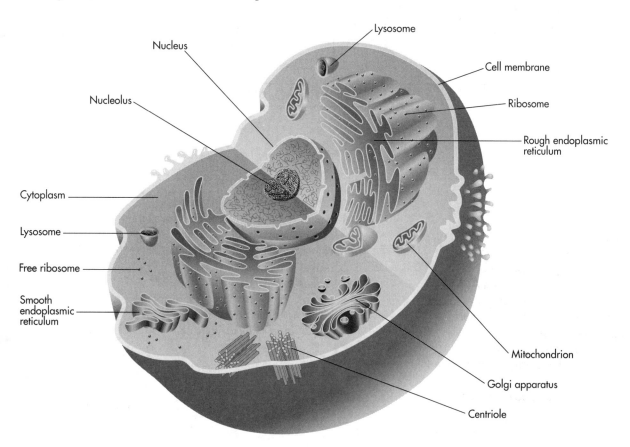

CROSSWORD PUZZLE

```
        ¹N U C L E O L U S
         U
        ²C A N C E R
         L
³S E M I P E R M ⁴E A B L E
 A       U       U
 T       S       K           ⁵R
 U      ⁶P H A G O C Y T O S I S
 R    ⁷M  ⁸M     R           B    ⁹I
¹⁰A C T I V E    Y           O    N
 T    T   T      O           S    T
 I    O   A      T       ¹¹G L U C O S E
 O    C   P  ¹²V I R U S     M    R
 N    H   H      C           E    P
      O ¹³A T P                   H
      N   S            ¹⁴M        A
      D ¹⁵E X O C Y T O S I S     S
      R                T          E
   ¹⁶D I F F U S I O N O
      A            ¹⁷L Y S O S O M E
                       I
                       S
```

Across
1. make ribosomes
2. cells reproducing out of control
3. only some substances can cross
6. cell engulfing solid particles
10. _____ transport uses ATP
11. broken down during cellular respiration
12. hijacks cell in order to reproduce
13. high energy molecule
15. substance leaves cell in a vesicle
16. movement of substance from high to low concentration
17. vesicle containing powerful enzymes

Down
1. contains genetic information for cell
3. all binding sites full
4. cell with nucleus and organelles
5. makes protein
7. makes ATP
8. chromosomes line up in center of cell
9. cell is not dividing
14. cell division of eukaryotic cells

CONCEPT MAP

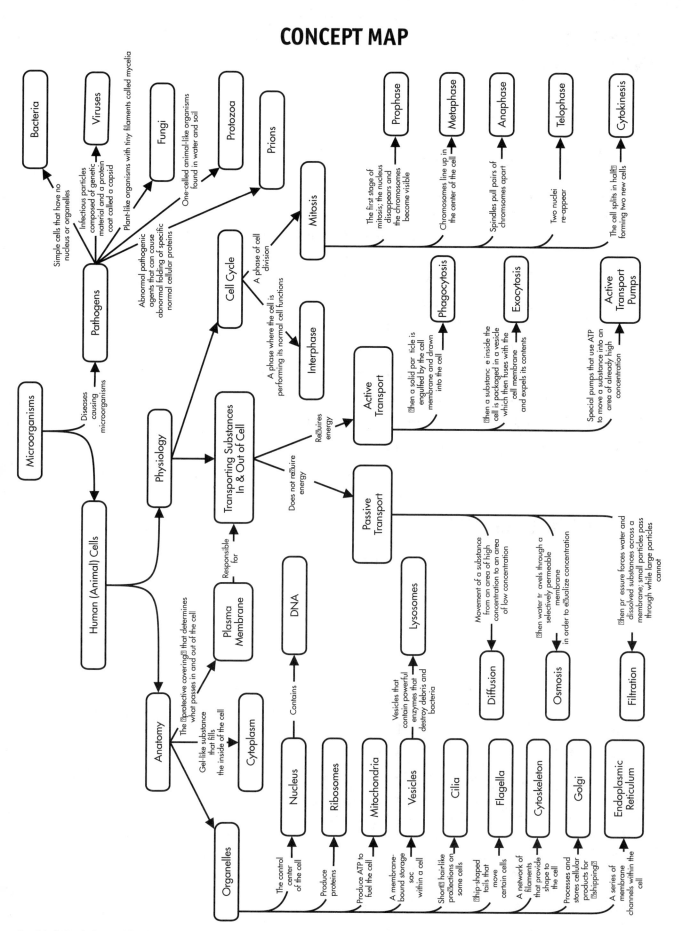

CHAPTER 5
ANSWER KEY

MEDICAL TERMINOLOGY REVIEW

1. Serous: A double-layered membrane that lines major cavities and covers the organs within the cavities
2. Mucous: A membrane that secretes mucus, usually lines cavities open to the outside of the body
3. Synovial: Membrane lining freely moving joints
4. Stratified: Multiple layers of cells, usually refers to epithelial tissue
5. Striated: Striped, usually refers to muscle fibers
6. Matrix: Extracellular material in tissues
7. Tissue: A collection of similar cells united in a common function
8. Organ: A collection of tissues united in a common function
9. System: A collection of organs sharing a common function
10. Vital: An organ that is necessary for life

MULTIPLE CHOICE

1. c
2. b
3. a
4. c
5. a
6. c
7. b
8. b
9. a
10. b
11. a
12. a
13. a
14. d
15. c
16. b
17. b
18. d
19. d
20. d
21. c
22. a
23. a
24. c
25. b

MATCHING EXERCISES

Set 1	Set 2	Set 3	Set 4
1. h	1. k	1. e	1. d
2. d	2. e	2. a	2. j
3. b	3. h	3. k	3. b
4. j	4. d	4. j	4. e
5. c	5. j	5. c	5. i
6. e	6. g	6. b	6. h
7. g	7. l	7. g	7. a
8. a	8. c	8. d	8. g
9. i	9. i	9. i	9. c
10. f	10. b	10. h	10. f

FILL IN THE BLANK

1. serous
2. heart
3. neuroglia
4. endocrine
5. digestive
6. cardiovascular
7. nervous and sensory
8. shape
9. Neuroglia
10. epithelial
11. connective
12. striated
13. synovial
14. connective
15. lymphatic
16. wound healing
17. adipose
18. thorax
19. Nervous or cardiac muscle
20. matrix
21. cartilage
22. matrix
23. regenerative
24. epithelium
25. pluripotent

SHORT ANSWER

1. The four types of tissue are epithelial, connective, muscle, and nervous. Epithelial tissue covers and lines much of the body and covers many parts found in the body. Connective tissue holds things together and provides structure and support. Muscle tissue contracts and by doing so moves bone and moves substances throughout and out of the body. Nervous tissue conducts impulses.

2. Cardiac muscle is found in the walls of the heart. It is striated, branched, and has only one nucleus per cell. Skeletal muscle is found attached to bone. It is striated, multinucleate, and has cylindrical cells. Smooth muscle lines hollow organs and vessels. It is not striated. Both cardiac and smooth muscles are involuntary, and skeletal muscle is voluntary.

3. Tissue repair or wound healing begins with inflammation and clotting if the injury is bleeding. Next, fibroblasts pull the edges of the wound together and make a delicate pink tissue. Then either regeneration (replacement with the original tissue) or fibrosis (scarring-replacement with collagen fibers) occurs.

4. Serous membranes are composed of visceral and parietal layers that reduce friction between different tissues and organs. The parietal layer lines cavities, and the visceral layer adheres to the organs. There is a potential space between the layers.

5. Both the endocrine and nervous systems control the activity of virtually all the body organs. The nervous system does it by electrical impulses, and the endocrine system does it by chemicals called hormones.

LABELING ACTIVITY

See Figure 5–1 in the textbook for comparison.

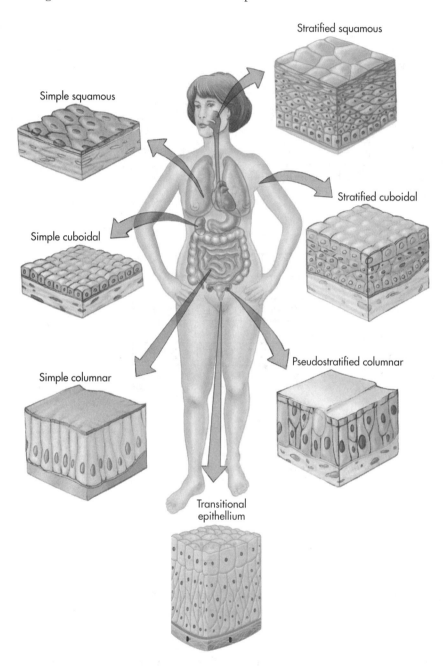

CROSSWORD PUZZLE

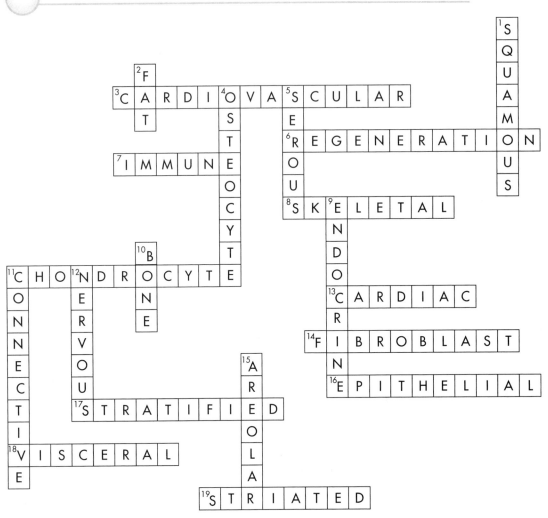

Across
- 3. the heart is part of the _____ system
- 6. wound is repaired by original tissue
- 7. this system fights infection
- 8. the _____ system makes red blood cells
- 11. cartilage cell
- 13. muscle with connections between cells
- 14. cell that repairs damaged tissue
- 16. _____ tissue has no extracellular matrix
- 17. tissue with more than one layer of cells
- 18. the _____ layer of the pericardium covers the heart surface
- 19. skeletal muscle is _____ muscle

Down
- 1. plate-like cells
- 2. common name for adipose tissue
- 4. mature bone cell
- 5. double layered membrane
- 9. this system controls the body by releasing hormones
- 10. cells in mineral matrix
- 11. tissue with extracellular matrix
- 12. this system contains the brain, spinal cord, nerves
- 15. web-like support tissue

Copyright © 2020 by Pearson Education, Inc.

CONCEPT MAP

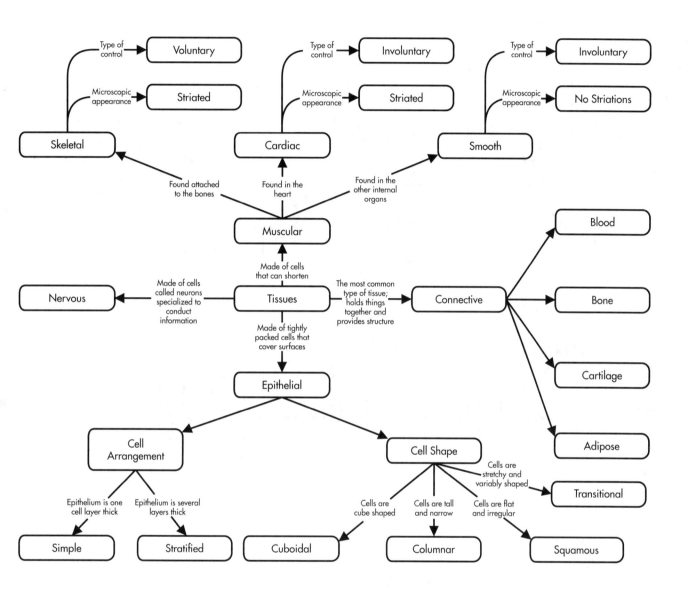

CONCEPT MAP

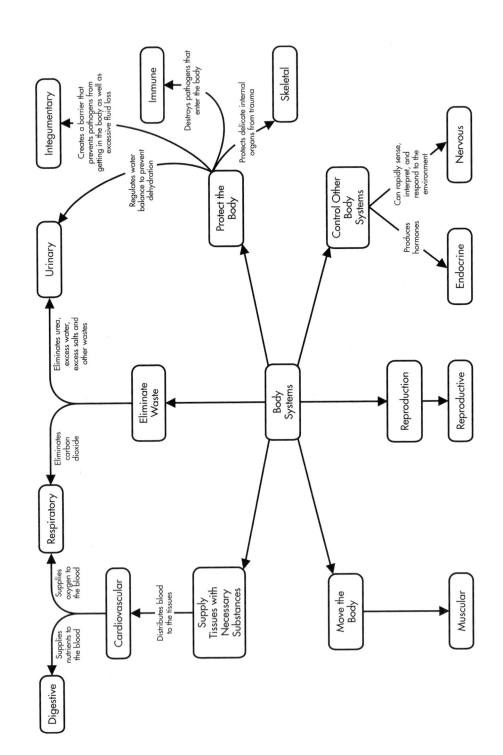

CHAPTER 6
ANSWER KEY

MEDICAL TERMINOLOGY REVIEW

1. Osteoporosis: Decreased bone density leading to porous bones
2. Arthritis: Joint inflammation
3. Ossification: Bone formation
4. Osteon: Fundamental unit of compact bone, cylinder of osteocytes surrounding central canal
5. Articulation: Where bones meet, joint
6. Ligament: Connective tissue that holds bones together
7. Tendon: Connective tissue that holds muscle to bone
8. Reduction: Bringing the ends of fractured bones into alignment
9. Sternum: Medial bone of the anterior thorax to which the clavicle and ribs are attached; also called the breastbone
10. Comminuted fracture: Broken bone in which the bone is crushed into fragments or splinters

MULTIPLE CHOICE

1. c
2. b
3. a
4. c
5. e
6. b
7. b
8. a
9. c
10. b
11. a
12. d
13. c
14. b
15. d
16. a
17. a
18. b
19. a
20. d
21. c
22. c
23. a
24. c
25. a

MATCHING EXERCISES

Set 1	Set 2	Set 3	Set 4
1. m	1. j	1. d	1. a
2. c	2. g	2. c	2. f
3. j	3. c	3. e	3. d
4. i	4. i	4. j	4. j
5. e	5. f	5. a	5. g
6. g	6. a	6. g	6. c
7. d	7. h	7. i	7. b
8. k	8. b	8. h	8. h
9. h	9. e	9. b	9. i
10. b	10. d	10. f	10. e

FILL IN THE BLANK

1. osteoporosis
2. congenital
3. cervical/lumbar
4. monocytes
5. plantar flex
6. extension
7. mandible
8. body
9. vertebrocostal
10. hinge
11. endochondral ossification
12. arthritis
13. 206
14. comminuted
15. osteoclasts
16. remodeling
17. perforating
18. cartilage
19. calcium and phosphorus
20. Compact
21. ulna and radius
22. osteoclast
23. Suture lines
24. trabeculae
25. Spongy bone

SHORT ANSWER

1. The functions of the skeleton are to provide a framework, produce blood cells, protect organs, serve as a warehouse for mineral storage, and move with the assistance of the muscles.

2. The four types of bones are the flat, long, short, and irregular. Flat bones are platelike and include the sternum, ribs, and cranium. Long bones are longer than they are wide, and examples include bones of the arms and legs. Short bones are equal in width and length and found in the ankle and wrist. Irregular bones are odd-shaped bones such as the hip and vertebrae.

3. The main function of the periosteum is to cover the bone. The periosteum contains the blood vessels, nerves, and lymph that serve the bone itself. It also acts as an anchor for ligaments and tendons.

4. A ligament is a fibrous tissue connecting bone to bone usually over a joint. A tendon attaches muscle to bone.

5. Intramembranous ossification occurs when bone develops between two sheets composed of fibrous connective tissue. Cells from connective tissue turn into osteoblasts and form a matrix that is similar to the trabeculae of spongy bone. The majority of human bones are created through endochondral ossification in which shaped cartilage is replaced by bone. Periosteum surrounds the diaphysis of the cartilage bone as the cartilage itself begins to break down. Osteoblasts come into this region and create spongy bone in an area that is then called the primary ossification center. Meanwhile, other osteoblasts begin to form compact bone under the periosteum. Here is where the osteoclasts come into play. Their job is to break down the spongy bone of the diaphysis to create the medullary cavity. After birth, the epiphyses on the long bones continue to grow. However, shortly after birth, secondary ossification of this area begins with spongy bone forming and not breaking down.

LABELING ACTIVITY

See Figure 6–3 in the textbook for comparison.

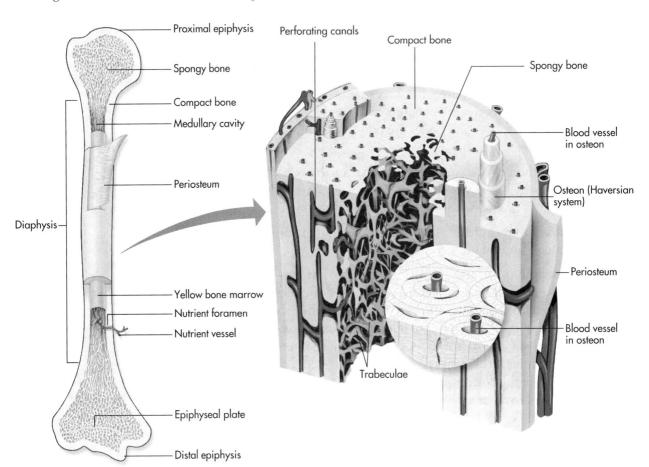

CROSSWORD PUZZLE

```
      ¹O ²S  T  ³E  O  B  L  A  ⁴T
         K     P              A
         U     I              R          ⁵G
         L     P         ⁶O  S  T  ⁷E  O  C  L  A  S  ⁸T
         L     ⁹H  I  N  G  E     A        S           E
               Y              A        T     D        N
¹⁰C  A  R ¹¹P  A  L  S        L        E     I        D
  A        E        I    ¹²P  S        O     N        O
  R        R      ¹³S  Y  N  O  V  I  A ¹⁴L N        N
  T        I        I        V        I
  I        O        A        O        G
  L      ¹⁵S  T  E ¹⁶R  N  U  M        T     A
  A        T        I                        M     ¹⁷H
  G        E        B                 ¹⁸F  E  M  U  R
  E        U        S                        N     M
           M                                 T     E
                                                   R
                                                   U
                                 ¹⁹D  I  A  P  H  Y  S  I  S
```

Across

1. cell which makes bone
6. cell which tears down bone
9. a joint which only flexes and extends
10. wrist bones
13. membrane lining freely moving joints
15. breastbone
18. thigh bone
19. shaft of long bone

Down

2. bones made by intramembranous ossification
3. expanded end of long bone
4. ankle bones
5. joint in wrist
7. a cylinder of bone
8. _____ attaches muscle to bone
10. the early embryonic skeleton is made of this tissue
11. covers bone
12. joint which can only rotate
14. _____ attaches bone to bone
16. these bones in the thoracic cage are flat bones
17. upper arm bone

CONCEPT MAP

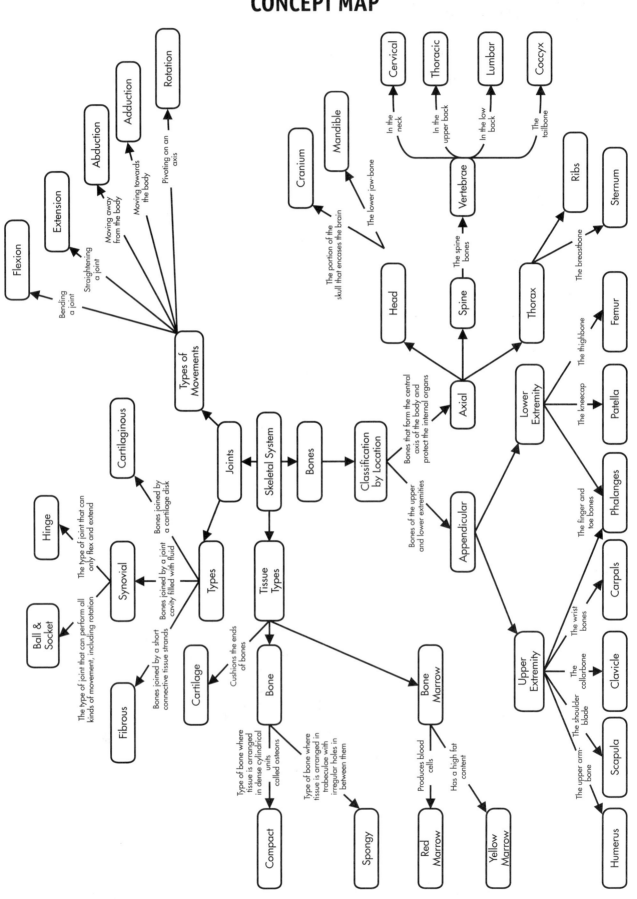

CHAPTER 7
ANSWER KEY

MEDICAL TERMINOLOGY REVIEW

1. Sprain: Ligament injury
2. Myalgia: Muscle pain or tenderness
3. Paralysis: Inability to control voluntary movements
4. Hypertrophy: Increase in muscle diameter and strength
5. Atrophy: Decrease in muscle size; muscle wasting
6. Tonus: Partial muscle contraction
7. Spasm: Sudden, severe muscle contraction
8. Muscular dystrophy: Inherited disorder that causes deterioration of muscle fibers; most common in boys
9. Electromyogram: Recording of electrical activity of a muscle
10. Strain: Injury or tear to tendon or muscle

MULTIPLE CHOICE

1. a
2. b
3. b
4. a
5. c
6. d
7. a
8. a
9. c
10. b
11. c
12. c
13. c
14. a
15. d
16. c
17. c
18. a
19. c
20. d
21. c
22. b
23. c
24. d
25. d

MATCHING EXERCISES

Set 1	Set 2	Set 3	Set 4
1. h	1. e	1. h	1. d
2. e	2. i	2. i	2. g
3. f	3. c	3. a	3. e
4. i	4. f	4. b	4. j
5. b	5. d	5. c	5. b
6. c	6. h	6. e	6. f
7. a	7. g	7. d	7. c
8. j	8. j	8. g	8. a
9. d	9. b	9. k	9. h
10. g	10. a	10. f	10. i

FILL IN THE BLANK

1. intercalated discs
2. peristalsis
3. triceps brachii
4. glycogen
5. sarcomere
6. acetylcholine
7. Z-lines
8. quadriceps
9. synergists
10. visceral
11. heart
12. tendon
13. shape
14. arm
15. ATP and calcium
16. actin
17. shin splints
18. tetanus
19. ataxia
20. ligament
21. tendonitis
22. sodium
23. calcium
24. hamstrings
25. Achilles (calcaneal)

Copyright © 2020 by Pearson Education, Inc.

SHORT ANSWER

1. Skeletal muscles can be named based on their size, shape, location, attachment location, number of attachments, action, and fiber direction. A combination of rules may also be used.

2. Acetylcholine, a neurotransmitter, is released from a neuron. Acetylcholine binds to muscle and causes sodium channels to open. Sodium flows into the muscle fiber, and the fiber becomes excited. The excitement of the muscle fiber causes calcium to be released into the cytoplasm from the sarcoplasmic reticulum. The calcium allows the forming of cross-bridges between myosin heads and actin myofilaments. ATP is used up, allowing cross-bridges to break and reform, pulling the actin myofilaments closer together as they slide along the myosin myofilaments. The sarcomere shortens. Many shortened sarcomeres results in shortening of many muscle fibers. This is muscle contraction. Finally, acetylcholinesterase degrades acetylcholine so the muscle can relax.

3. Muscle, like all tissue, needs fuel in the form of nutrients and oxygen to survive and function. The body stores a carbohydrate called glycogen in the muscle. When needed, the muscle can convert glycogen to glucose, which releases energy for the muscle to function. Muscles with very high demands (such as leg muscles) also store fat and use it as energy. The higher-demand muscles not only use fat as an energy source but they also have a much richer blood supply than do less demanding muscles.

4. The origin is the stationary attachment. The insertion moves. The action, then, occurs when the insertion moves toward the origin.

5. Skeletal muscles are voluntary muscles that usually attach to bone. Smooth muscles are involuntary muscles found in organ walls, blood vessel walls, and airways. Cardiac muscle is involuntary and found as one of the layers surrounding the heart.

LABELING ACTIVITY

See Figure 7–2 in the textbook for comparison.

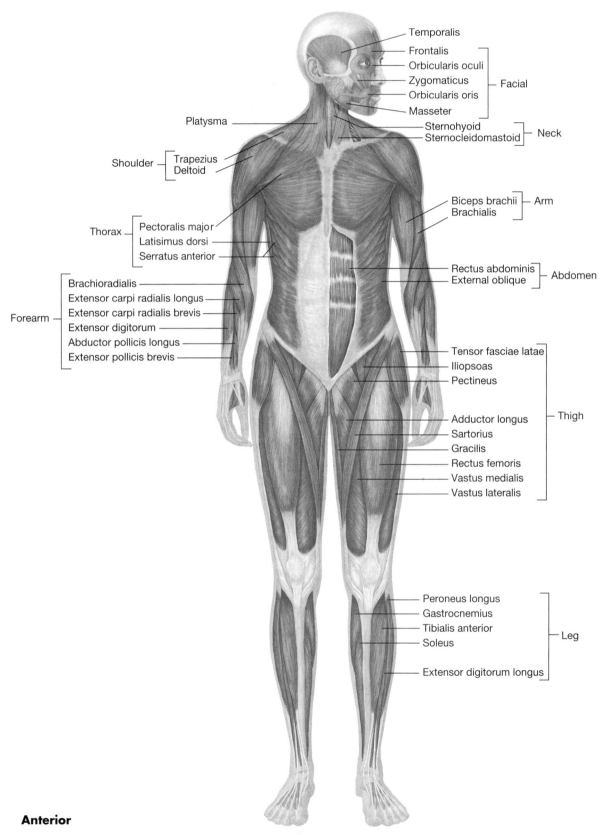

Anterior

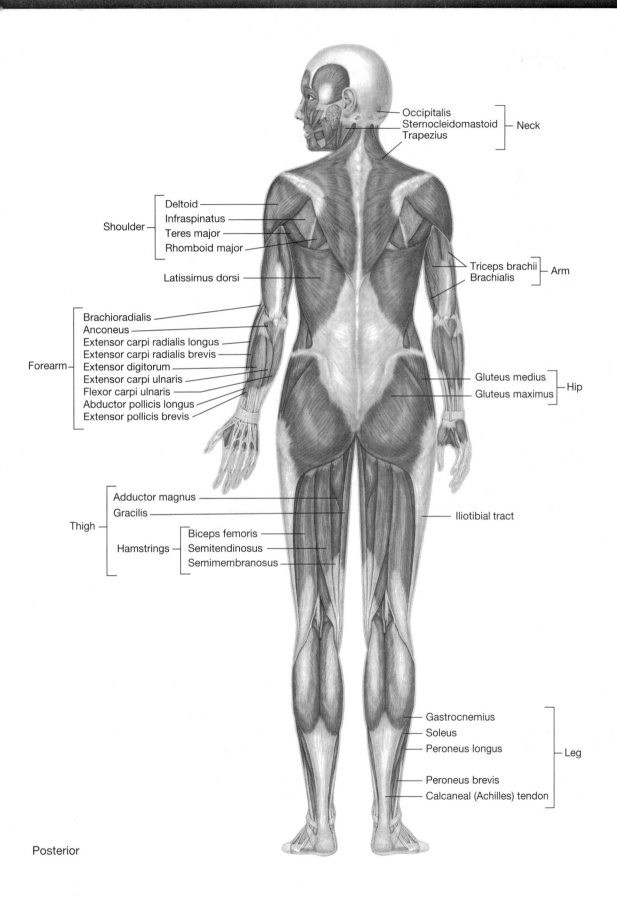

Posterior

CROSSWORD PUZZLE

Across

2. neurotransmitter that excites skeletal muscle
5. thin filament
9. cylindrical subdivision of muscle fiber
10. spinning on axis
11. prime movement of muscle
12. movement toward center
15. sheet-like muscle attachments
16. fundamental contractile unit of muscle

Down

1. decreased joint angle
2. movement away from center
3. stationary attachments
4. Increased joint angle
6. ion necessary for cross-bridge formation
7. aids primary mover
8. the _____ reticulum stores calcium
9. The medical name for a muscle cell
11. opposes the prime mover
12. prime mover
13. mobile muscle attachments
14. thick filament

CONCEPT MAP

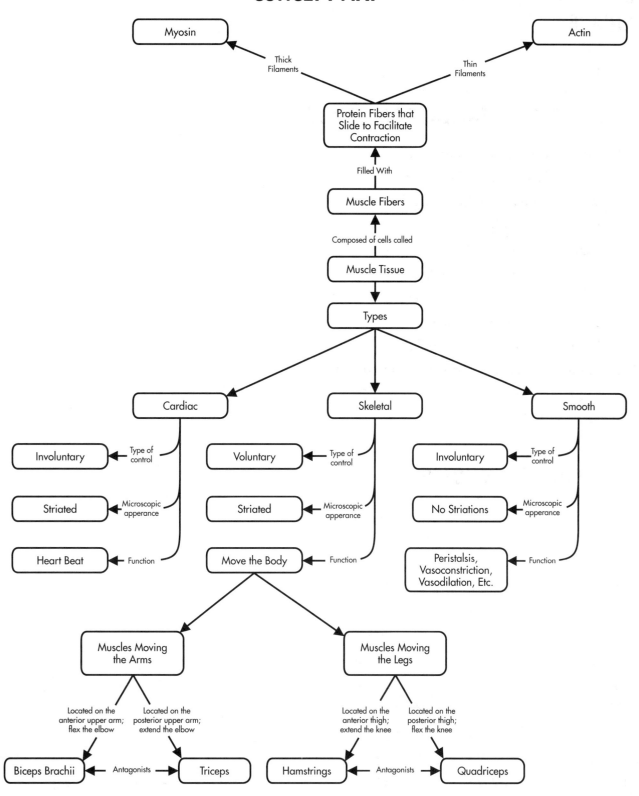

CHAPTER 8
ANSWER KEY

MEDICAL TERMINOLOGY REVIEW

1. Macule: Discolored spot on skin
2. Pustule: Elevated pus-filled lesion
3. Wheal: Raised, often itchy spot
4. Ulcer: Eating away of the skin
5. Papule: Solid, elevated area on skin
6. Crust: Dry brown, green, red, or yellow area
7. Keloid: A mass of scar tissue that has a raised, firm, irregular shape
8. Scale: Thin, dry, flaky epidermis
9. Vesicle: Small sac filled with fluid
10. Fissure: Crack or slit that reaches into dermis

MULTIPLE CHOICE

1. d
2. c
3. c
4. a
5. d
6. c
7. b
8. c
9. a
10. a
11. a
12. b
13. d
14. d
15. b
16. a
17. a
18. c
19. c
20. a
21. c
22. a
23. c
24. a
25. b

MATCHING EXERCISES

Set 1	Set 2	Set 3	Set 4
1. a	1. g	1. b	1. b
2. g	2. h	2. j	2. e
3. h	3. d	3. e	3. h
4. d	4. j	4. g	4. j
5. e	5. i	5. c	5. a
6. j	6. c	6. a	6. c
7. i	7. a	7. h	7. g
8. f	8. e	8. i	8. i
9. c	9. b	9. f	9. f
10. b	10. f	10. d	10. d

FILL IN THE BLANK

1. collagenous and elastic
2. melanoma
3. herpes zoster
4. arrector pili
5. stratum corneum
6. pustule
7. 12
8. 3
9. hematoma
10. sebum
11. third
12. 63
13. root
14. melanin
15. bilirubin
16. lesion
17. Albinism
18. shingles
19. skin
20. dermis
21. subcutaneous
22. depth, extent
23. hives
24. decubitus
25. vitamin D production, protection against fluid loss, protection against UV radiation, temperature regulation, sensory input

SHORT ANSWER

1. Epidermal cells are born in the stratum germinativum, a deeper region located in the stratum basale. As the cell moves toward the surface (stratum corneum), it dies and fills with the protein keratin. By the time the cell is in the stratum corneum, it is dead.

2. Basal cell carcinoma usually spreads locally and can usually be successfully treated. Squamous cell carcinoma may develop deeper into tissue but rarely spreads to other tissue. Malignant melanoma develops deep in the skin and can spread throughout the body to various organs.

3. Pressure ulcers (bedsores, decubitus ulcers) are a result of a lack of blood flow to skin that has had pressure applied to a bony prominence.

4. Skin acts as storage for fatty tissue necessary for energy, keeps us from drying out, provides sensory impulse, regulates body temperature, and protects from disease producing pathogens.

5. Burns are classified by depth and extent. Depth is described by degrees. First-degree burns affect only the epidermis. Second-degree burns affect both the epidermis and the dermis. Third- and fourth-degree burns burn fully through the skin. Extent is expressed as percent of surface burned using the rule of nines.

LABELING ACTIVITY

See Figure 8–1 in the textbook for comparison.

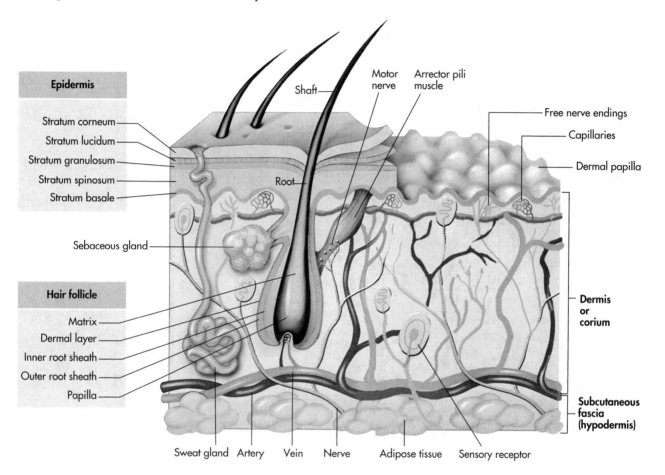

CROSSWORD PUZZLE

```
            ¹D           ²H
 ³S T R A T U M ⁴C O R N E U ⁵M       A       ⁶M
   W           U           P   ⁷E C C R I N E
   ⁸K E R ⁹A T I N         T       L     F     L
     A   R                 H       A     O     A
     T   R                         N     L     N
         E         ¹⁰D E R M I ¹¹S  I     L     O
         C             O       T    N     I     C
         T             U       R          C     Y
         O             S       A          L     T
  ¹²H Y ¹³P O D E R M I S       T          E     E
     E    P                    U
     R   ¹⁴V I T ¹⁵A M I ¹⁶N D  M
     F    L       P       I    B
     U    I       O       N    A
     S            C       E   ¹⁷S E B A C E O U ¹⁸S
     I            R       S    A                 K
     O            I            L                 I
     N            N                              N
                 ¹⁹E P I D E R M I S
```

Across

3. the outer layer of dead epidermal cells
7. sweat glands which help regulate body temperature
8. hardened protein found in hair and nails
10. layer of skin with connective tissue and accessory structures
12. deepest skin layer
14. made when skin is exposed to sunlight (2 words)
17. _____ glands secrete oil
19. surface layer of skin

Down

1. Burns can be categorized by _____ and extent
2. hair grows from cells in the _____ (2 words)
3. secreted when body temperature rises
4. pertaining to skin
5. dark skin pigment
6. melanoma is cancer of this cell
9. contraction of this muscle makes hair stand on end (2 words)
11. epidermal cells are born here
13. _____ is monitored using the nails
15. secretes a sexual attractant
16. extent of burn injury is determined using rule of _____
18. medical term is integument

CONCEPT MAP

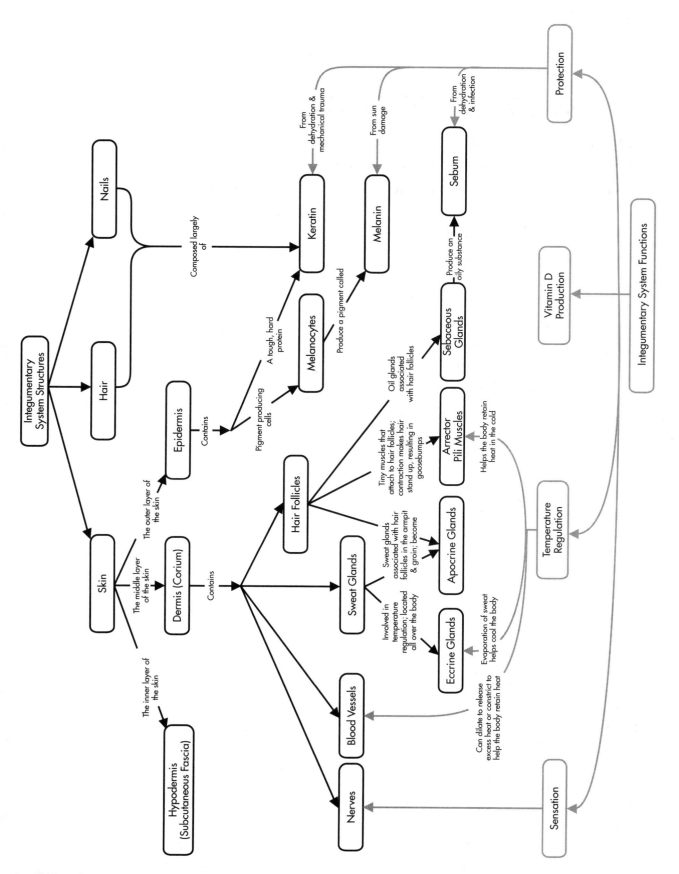

CHAPTER 9
ANSWER KEY

MEDICAL TERMINOLOGY REVIEW

1. Neuropathy: decrease in function or peripheral nerves
2. Paralysis: inability to control voluntary movements
3. Spinal cord injury: damage to the spinal cord caused by disease or injury
4. Carpal tunnel syndrome: inflammation and swelling of the tendon sheaths surrounding the flexor tendon of the palm
5. Multiple sclerosis: autoimmune destruction of myelin in the CNS
6. Guillain-Barré syndrome: Destruction of myelin in the peripheral nervous system, characterized by rapid onset ascending paralysis
7. Meningitis: Infection of the membranes surrounding the CNS
8. Myasthenia gravis: Autoimmune attack on acetylcholine receptors in the neuromuscular junction
9. Paraplegia: Paralysis in the lower limbs
10. Quadriplegia: Paralysis in all four limbs

MULTIPLE CHOICE

1. b
2. b
3. c
4. b
5. d
6. a
7. c
8. c
9. d
10. d
11. a
12. a
13. c
14. b
15. a
16. c
17. a
18. b
19. a
20. b
21. c
22. a
23. c
24. c
25. c

MATCHING EXERCISES

Set 1	Set 2	Set 3	Set 4
1. i	1. d	1. d	1. e
2. j	2. b	2. e	2. a
3. d	3. c	3. g	3. g
4. c	4. g	4. h	4. j
5. f	5. i	5. f	5. b
6. k	6. h	6. c	6. c
7. b	7. k	7. i	7. h
8. e	8. j	8. a	8. f
9. h	9. f	9. b	9. i
10. g	10. e	10. j	10. d

FILL IN THE BLANK

1. resting, digesting
2. synapse
3. neurotransmitters
4. ventral (or anterior)/dorsal (or posterior)/lateral
5. epidural/dura mater
6. anterior median fissure/posterior median sulcus
7. conus medullaris
8. dorsal/ventral
9. reflex
10. median
11. vesicles
12. meninges
13. depolarized
14. sodium
15. multiple sclerosis
16. phrenic
17. sensory
18. dorsal column
19. ventral horn
20. thoracic
21. shock absorber
22. C4
23. hyperpolarized
24. myelin
25. central canal

SHORT ANSWER

1. Myelin is a lipid, so ions cannot cross. Thus the only part of an axon that can depolarize are the nodes of Ranvier. So in a myelinated axon, the AP hops from node to node, which is faster than conduction in an unmyelinated axon, which must depolarize along the entire length.

2. When that cell is stimulated (excited), voltage gated sodium channels in the cell membrane spring open. Sodium ions (Na^+) travel into the cell, making the cell more positive. A cell that is more positive than at rest is called depolarized. The gates on the sodium channels shut, and then they open. Potassium (K^+), which is also positive, leaves the cell, taking its positive charges with it. The inside of the cell becomes more negative again, eventually returning to rest. This is repolarization. Sometimes a cell overshoots and becomes more negative than when it is at rest. Then the cell is hyperpolarized. Eventually, the cell will return to resting.

3. The terminal depolarizes, calcium channels open, and calcium rushes in. The calcium coming in causes vesicles filled with neurotransmitter to fuse to the membrane. Neurotransmitter is released (via exocytosis) into the synapse and diffuses across. Neurotransmitter binds to the postsynaptic cell, causing a permeability change. Then cleanup occurs.

4. A reflex consists of a sensory neuron, spinal nerve, association neuron, and motor neuron.

5. Action potential is all-in-one; once it starts, it will always finish and will always be the same size, whereas the graded potentials vary in size.

LABELING ACTIVITY

See Figure 5–10 in the textbook for comparison.

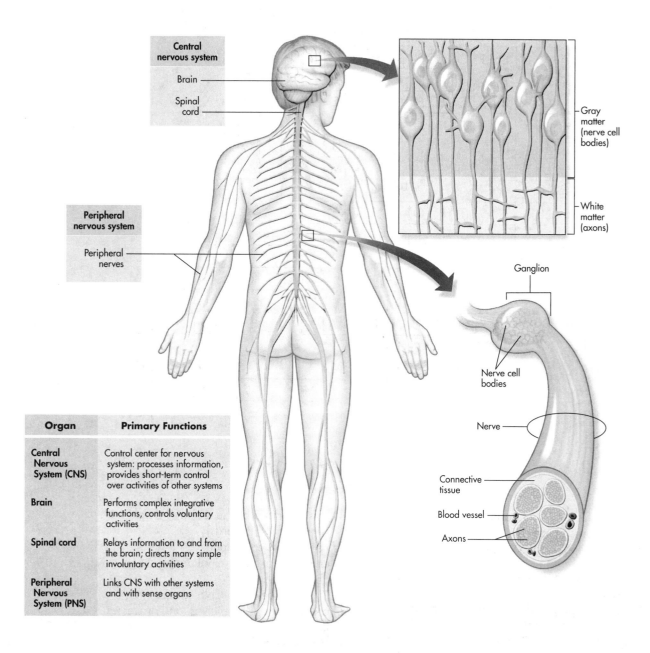

CROSSWORD PUZZLE

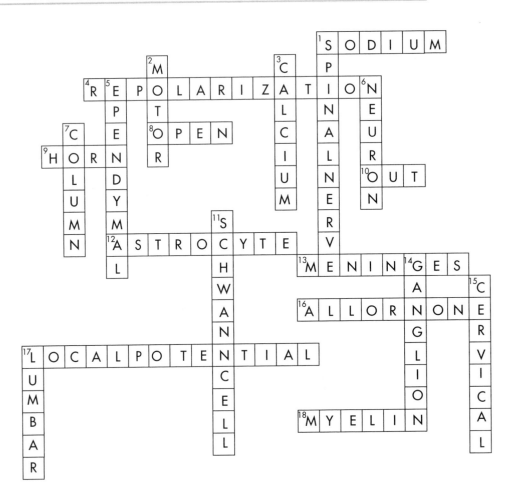

Across
1. this ion is important during depolarization
4. cell returns to resting
8. during repolarization, potassium channels _____
9. motor neurons in the spinal cord are in the ventral _____
10. during hyperpolarization, potassium moves _____ of the cell
12. general support cell for CNS
13. dura mater, arachnoid mater, and pia mater
16. action potentials do not change size, they are _____ (3 words)
17. change in cell charge that is proportional to stimulus (2 words)
18. made by oligodendrocytes

Down
1. This is formed by the fusion of dorsal and ventral roots (2 words)
2. nervous system output
3. enters the axon terminal during depolarization
5. _____ cells line CNS cavities
6. cell which sends, receives, and processes information
7. runs up and down the spinal cord
11. makes myelin for PNS (2 words)
14. collection of neurons outside CNS
15. the phrenic nerve projects from the _____ spinal cord
17. lower back

CONCEPT MAP

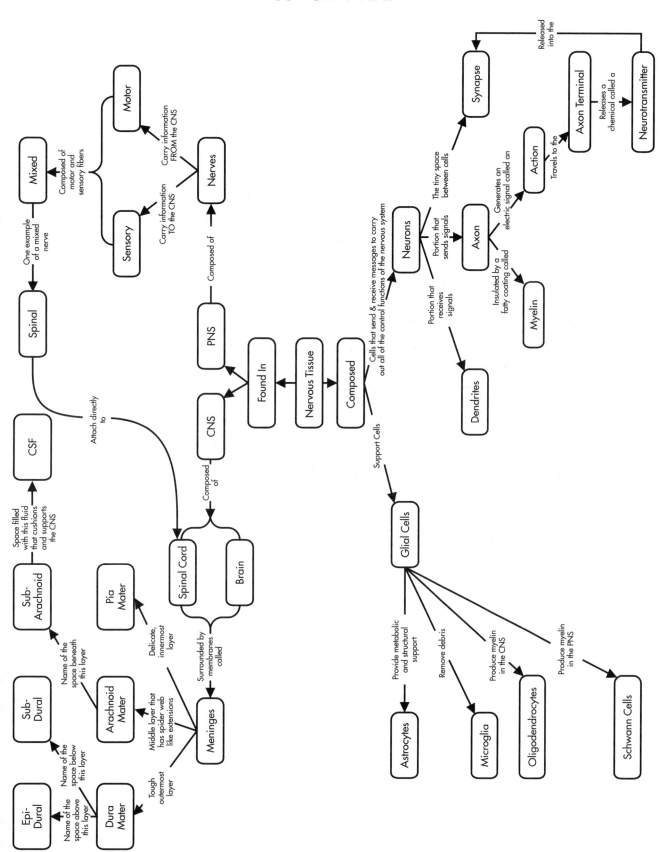

CHAPTER 10
ANSWER KEY

MEDICAL TERMINOLOGY REVIEW

1. Spastic: Type of paralysis characterized by hyperreflexia and rigid muscles
2. Flaccid: Type of paralysis characterized by decreased reflexes and floppy muscles
3. Cerebral palsy: Nonprogressive congenital movement disorder
4. Cerebral vascular accident: Also known as a CVA, stroke, brain damage caused by interruption of blood flow to brain tissue either due to hemorrhage or blood clot
5. Coma: Unconsciousness without response to stimuli
6. Traumatic brain injury: Abbreviated as TBI; occurs when force is applied to the skull causing brain damage.
7. Huntington's disease: Progressive inherited disorder that leads to dementia and movement disorders
8. Parkinson's disease: Progressive loss of motor coordination due to destruction of basal nuclei
9. Hydrocephalus: Accumulation of CSF in ventricles, caused by overproduction, blockage, or decreased reabsorption
10. Concussion: A mild brain injury that may damage brain tissue, depending on the level of severity.

MULTIPLE CHOICE

1. a
2. a
3. c
4. b
5. d
6. d
7. c
8. a
9. b
10. b
11. b
12. c
13. b
14. d
15. b
16. b
17. b
18. a
19. d
20. a
21. d
22. c
23. a
24. c
25. a

MATCHING EXERCISES

Set 1
1. e
2. k
3. h
4. l
5. j
6. a
7. d
8. i
9. c
10. b

Set 2
1. i
2. l
3. j
4. k
5. d
6. g
7. b
8. c
9. h
10. f

Set 3
1. d
2. i
3. f
4. h
5. e
6. b
7. a
8. g
9. c
10. j

Set 4
1. f
2. d
3. j
4. i
5. a
6. h
7. b
8. c
9. g
10. e

FILL IN THE BLANK

1. cerebrum/brain stem/cerebellum
2. longitudinal
3. gyri
4. vagus/glossopharyngeal
5. vision
6. lateral sulcus
7. midbrain
8. cortex
9. temporal lobe
10. cerebral spinal fluid
11. spinocerebellar
12. adrenal
13. reticular formation
14. parasympathetic
15. motor
16. hydrocephalus
17. Transient ischemic attacks (TIAs)
18. Huntington's disease
19. left
20. cerebellum
21. nuclei
22. ganglion
23. brain stem
24. association
25. subarachnoid

SHORT ANSWER

1. The left side of the body is controlled by the right side of the cerebral cortex, and the right side of the body is controlled by the left brain.

2. Subcortical structures, such as the thalamus, basal nuclei, and cerebellum act as coordination centers for the motor system. The indirect spinal cord pathways, which fine-tune motor activity, project from the subcortical structures.

3. The purpose of convolutions is to increase the surface area of the brain so more neurons can be packed into a smaller space.

4. All 31 pairs of spinal nerves are mixed (motor and sensory). There are only 12 pairs of cranial nerves and not all are mixed. Some are mostly motor, such as the trochlear nerve, and some are mostly sensory, such as the olfactory nerve.

5. Both sympathetic and parasympathetic nervous systems have limited effects on the skeletal muscle. The autonomic nervous system controls involuntary muscles. The sympathetic nervous system increases heart rate and increases blood pressure by constricting blood vessels. The parasympathetic nervous system decreases heart rate, decreases blood pressure, and increases digestive activity.

LABELING ACTIVITY

See Figures 10–1 and 10–3 in the textbook for comparison.

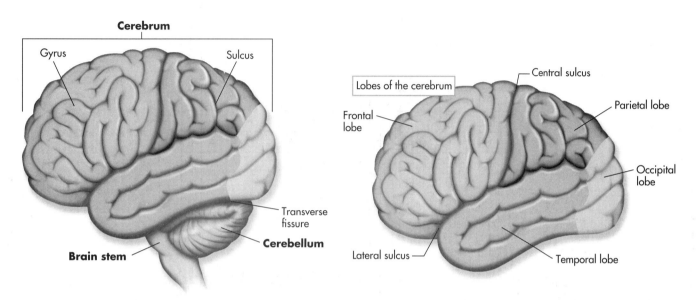

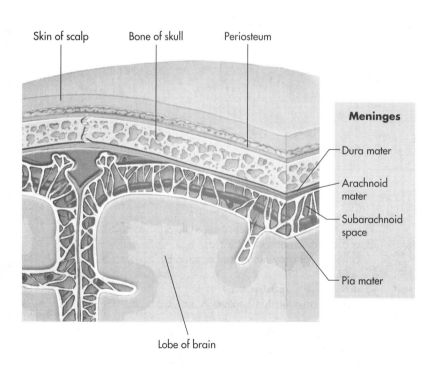

CROSSWORD PUZZLE

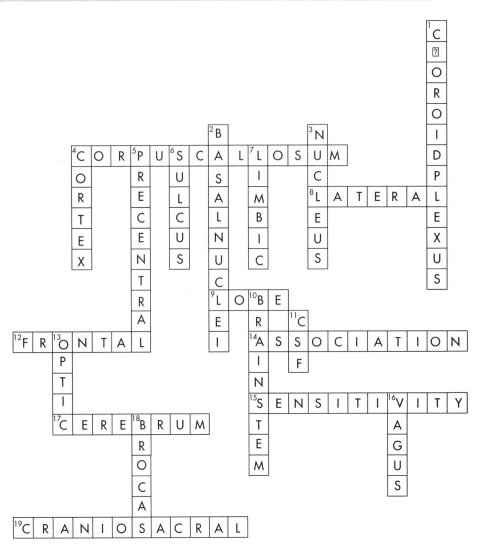

Across
- 4. connects left hemisphere to right (2 words)
- 8. this horn contains autonomic motor neurons
- 9. the occipital _____ contains the visual cortex
- 12. planning is accomplished in this lobe
- 14. areas which add meaning to sensation
- 15. map in the postcentral gyrus is determined by _____ of body
- 17. largest part of brain
- 19. location of parasympathetic preganglionic neurons

Down
- 1. tissue which makes cerebrospinal fluid (2 words)
- 2. coordination network (2 words)
- 3. collection of gray matter surrounded by white
- 4. outer layer of gray matter
- 5. a motor homunculus is found in the _____ gyrus
- 6. frontal and parietal lobes are separated by the central _____
- 7. the _____ system controls emotion, mood and memory
- 10. medulla oblongata, pons, midbrain
- 11. abbreviation for fluid found in ventricles
- 13. cranial nerve II
- 16. cranial nerve which controls viscera
- 18. motor area for speech

CONCEPT MAP

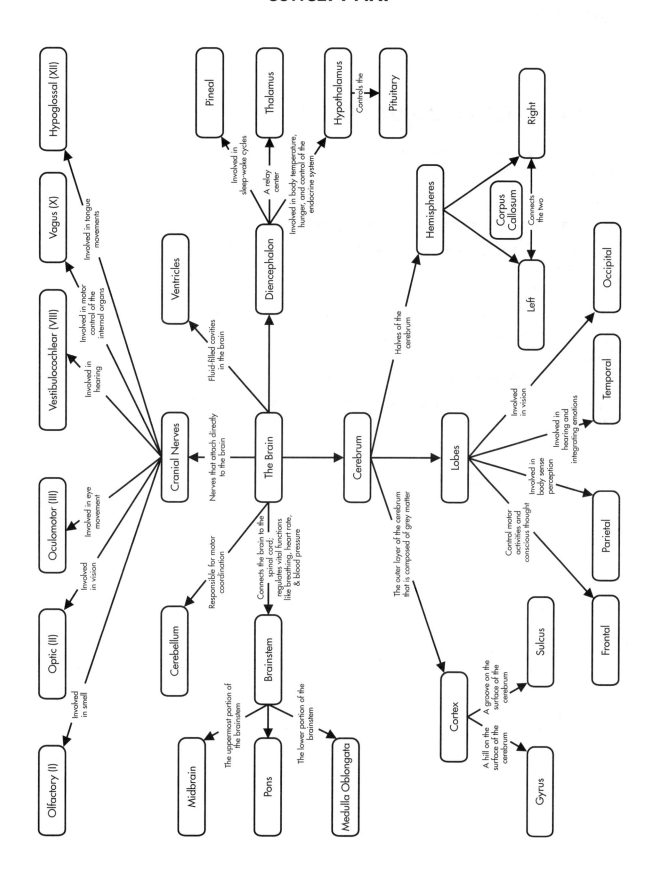

CHAPTER 11
ANSWER KEY

MEDICAL TERMINOLOGY REVIEW

1. Cataracts: Clouding of the lens of the eye causing decreased vision
2. Presbyopia: Age-related farsightedness
3. Myopia: Near-sightedness
4. Amblyopia: Lazy eye; one eye is excessively dominant
5. Glaucoma: Increased pressure inside the eyeball, which can lead to blindness if untreated
6. Vertigo: Feeling of dizziness or whirling in space
7. Otitis media: Middle ear infection usually caused by a bacteria or virus
8. Labyrinthitis: Inflammation of the inner ear usually is caused by high fevers
9. Phantom pain: Perception of pain or sensation in an amputated limb
10. Referred pain: Pain that originates in an internal organ, yet is felt in another region of the skin

MULTIPLE CHOICE

1. d
2. d
3. c
4. d
5. a
6. a
7. a
8. b
9. b
10. d
11. b
12. b
13. d
14. a
15. b
16. c
17. b
18. b
19. a
20. d
21. b
22. b
23. a
24. c
25. d

Copyright © 2020 by Pearson Education, Inc.

MATCHING EXERCISES

Set 1	Set 2	Set 3	Set 4
1. j	1. e	1. g	1. d
2. g	2. d	2. k	2. i
3. f	3. c	3. j	3. a
4. d	4. b	4. i	4. f
5. b	5. i	5. c	5. e
6. i	6. a	6. h	6. h
7. k	7. h	7. a	7. b
8. e	8. k	8. f	8. j
9. a	9. j	9. e	9. c
10. c	10. g	10. b	10. g

FILL IN THE BLANK

1. cochlea/temporal lobe
2. labyrinth
3. thresholds
4. lacrimal
5. iris
6. vitreous humor
7. bone
8. internal ear
9. auricle (pinna)
10. tympanic
11. perilymph, endolymph
12. pharynx
13. semicircular canals/cerebellum
14. cataracts
15. special
16. conjunctivitis
17. Smell
18. Taste
19. general
20. presbyopia
21. Vertigo
22. pain
23. labyrinth
24. organ of Corti
25. referred

SHORT ANSWER

1. Sound waves enter the external canal and vibrate the eardrum or tympanic membrane. The middle ear then amplifies the sound through the ossicles. The last ossicle (stapes) vibrates and causes a gentle pumping against the oval window membrane. This causes cochlear fluid to vibrate small hairlike neurons found in an area called the organ of Corti. As a result of the vibrating sensory cells (hairlike nerves), a nerve impulse is sent to the temporal lobe of the brain via cranial nerve VIII.

2. During adaptation there is continued sensory stimulation causing the sensors to desensitize or adapt. An example is when the temperature has not changed yet the body no longer feels the extreme hot or cold. It seems to be getting more neutral.

3. Accommodation combines changes in the size of the pupil and the lens curvature to make sure the image converges in the same place on the retina and therefore is properly focused.

4. The three layers of the eye are the sclera, the outermost layer commonly called the "white" of the eye; the middle layer, called the choroid, which contains the iris and pupil; and the deepest layer, called the retina, containing the nerve endings that receive and interpret the rays of light into what we see.

5. The three types of auditory conduction are sound, bone, and sensorineural conductions. Sound conduction is the vibration of the tympanic membrane by the actual sound waves. Bone conduction is the amplification of the waves by the ossicles (ear bones) or bones of skull. The last is the sensorineural conduction, the process by which the cochlear fluid vibrates the hairs to send nerve impulses to the temporal lobe of the brain where they are interpreted as sound.

LABELING ACTIVITIES

See Figure 11–2 in the textbook for comparison.

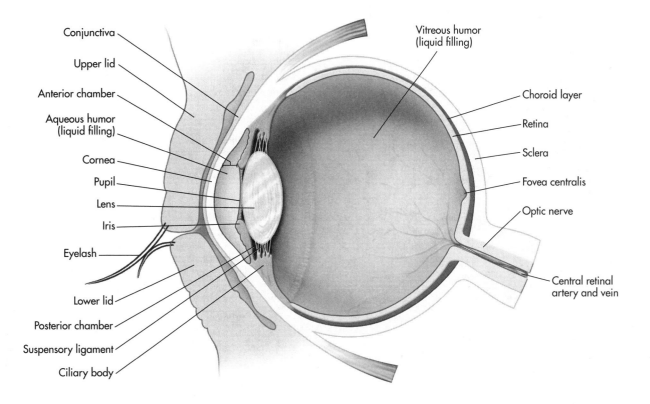

See Figure 11–3 in the textbook for comparison.

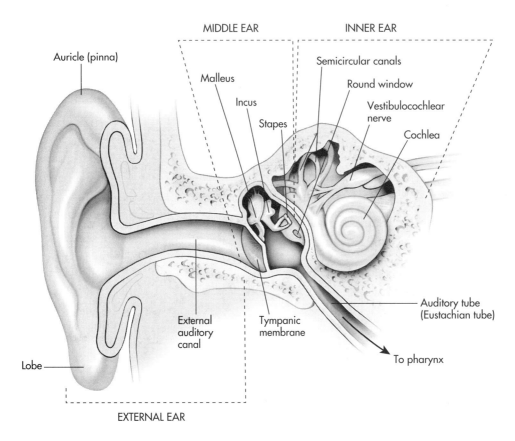

See Figure 11–9 in the textbook for comparison.

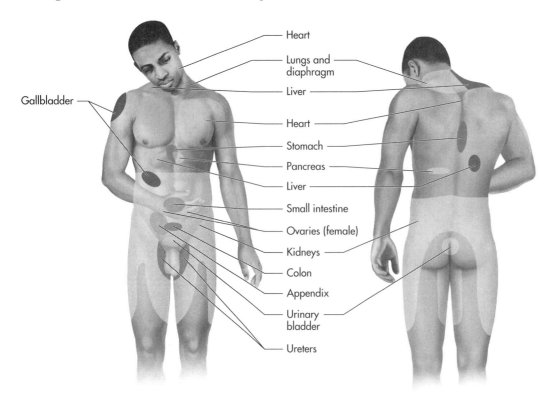

CROSSWORD PUZZLE

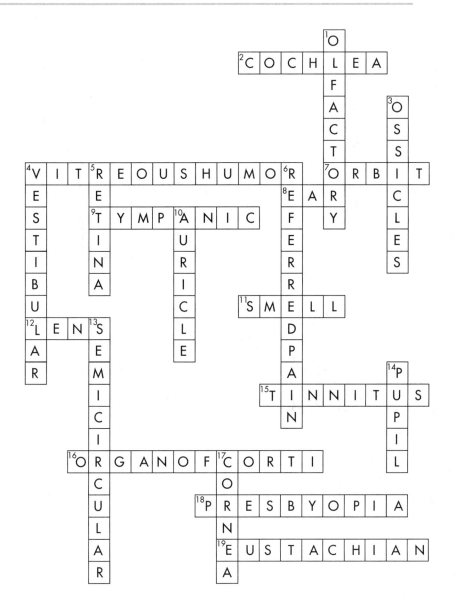

Across

2. structure containing sensory cells for hearing
4. _____ is the fluid filling the eyeball (2 words)
7. houses eyeball
8. organ of hearing
9. ear drum; _____ membrane
11. most important sense for interpreting taste
12. focuses light
15. ringing in the ears
16. auditory neurons embedded in this organ (3 words)
18. farsightedness associated with age
19. auditory or _____ tubes

Down

1. nerve which carries sense of smell
3. ear bones
4. balance sense
5. photoreceptor layer of eye
6. organ pain is _____ because it maps to body surface (2 words)
10. outer ear
13. _____ canals; vestibular sense
14. surrounds the iris
17. clear entrance to eye for light

Copyright © 2020 by Pearson Education, Inc.

CONCEPT MAP

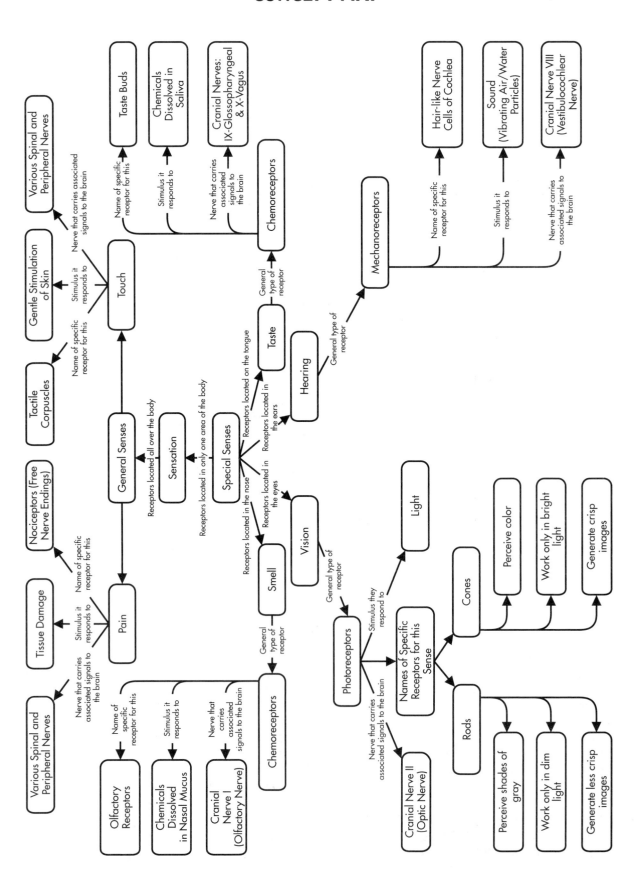

CHAPTER 12
ANSWER KEY

MEDICAL TERMINOLOGY REVIEW

1. Hypothyroidism: Decreased production of thyroid hormones
2. Hyperthyroidism: Increased production of thyroid hormones
3. Positive feedback: Mechanism that enhances hormone secretions
4. Negative feedback: A control mechanism that decreases hormone secretion as hormone levels rise
5. Endocrine: Type of secretions into the bloodstream that do not leave the body
6. Hormone: A chemical that is secreted into the bloodstream with effects on distant target cells
7. Steroids: Potent hormones that can pass through the cell membrane and interact directly with DNA
8. Cushing's syndrome: Oversecretion of cortisol typically caused by benign tumors; causes obesity, hypercholesterolemia, hypergylcemia
9. Diabetes mellitus: A disorder caused by decreased insulin secretion or insulin insensitivity, characterized by abnormally high blood glucose
10. Goiter: An enlarged thyroid gland that may be caused by thyroiditis, benign nodules, malignancies, or iodine deficiencies.

MULTIPLE CHOICE

1. d
2. c
3. a
4. b
5. d
6. d
7. a
8. c
9. b
10. b
11. a
12. d
13. a
14. b
15. a
16. d
17. a
18. d
19. b
20. a
21. d
22. c
23. b
24. c
25. b

Copyright © 2020 by Pearson Education, Inc.

MATCHING EXERCISES

Set 1	Set 2	Set 3	Set 4
1. f	1. f	1. b	1. g
2. c	2. b	2. i	2. j
3. i	3. k	3. c	3. f
4. d	4. g	4. g	4. a
5. g	5. i	5. h	5. d
6. h	6. c	6. a	6. h
7. e	7. d	7. j	7. c
8. j	8. j	8. d	8. e
9. a	9. h	9. f	9. b
10. b	10. a	10. e	10. i

FILL IN THE BLANK

1. oxytocin
2. adenohypophysis
3. thymus gland
4. insulin/glucagon
5. Addison's disease
6. thyroid-stimulating hormone (TSH)
7. prolactin/oxytocin
8. pituitary
9. estrogen secretion/sperm and egg production
10. antidiuretic hormone (ADH)
11. humoral/hormonal/neural
12. adrenal cortex
13. parathyroid
14. Hormones
15. progesterone
16. pheochromocytoma
17. pituitary
18. cortisol
19. acromegaly/gigantism
20. hypothyroidism
21. goiter
22. pancreas
23. glucagon
24. Glycogen
25. Paracrine

SHORT ANSWER

1. Endocrine glands secrete chemical messengers called hormones into the bloodstream, whereas exocrine glands secrete their substances into ducts that lead to either a lumen or to the outside of the body, such as digestive enzymes from the pancreas or sweat from the sweat glands (sudoriferous glands).

2. Mutual side effects of steroid abuse in both men and women include aggression, cardiovascular diseases, and increased cholesterol.

3. Alcohol suppresses a hormone called antidiuretic hormone (ADH), which is responsible for water uptake or water reabsorption in the kidney. If suppressed, it allows excessive water to be excreted rather than reabsorbed.

4. Humoral pertains to body fluids or substances. Humoral control controls hormones by monitoring body fluids such as blood, and responding accordingly via negative feedback.

5. Steroids and thyroid hormones are particularly powerful because they can bind to sites inside cells (intracellular sites). These hormones, which can pass through the cell membrane, can interact directly with the cell's DNA to change cell activity. Steroids and thyroid hormones are carefully regulated by the body because of their ability, even in very small amounts, to control target cells.

LABELING ACTIVITY

See Figure 5–11 in the textbook for comparison.

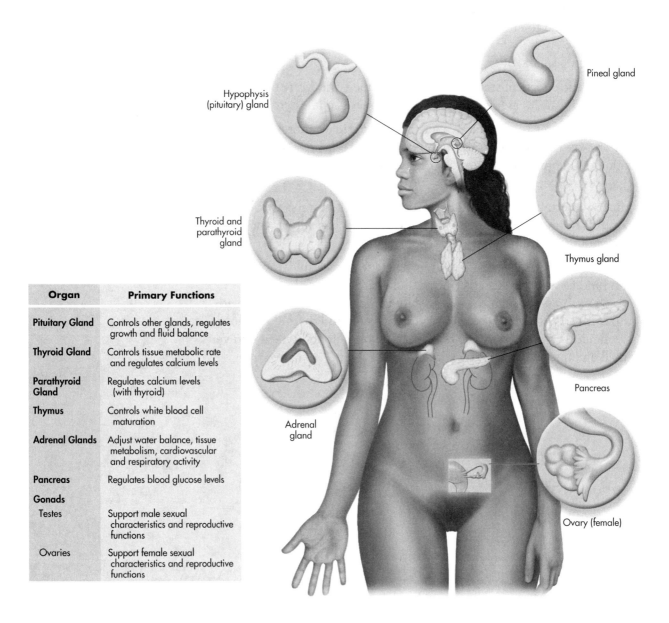

Organ	Primary Functions
Pituitary Gland	Controls other glands, regulates growth and fluid balance
Thyroid Gland	Controls tissue metabolic rate and regulates calcium levels
Parathyroid Gland	Regulates calcium levels (with thyroid)
Thymus	Controls white blood cell maturation
Adrenal Glands	Adjust water balance, tissue metabolism, cardiovascular and respiratory activity
Pancreas	Regulates blood glucose levels
Gonads	
Testes	Support male sexual characteristics and reproductive functions
Ovaries	Support female sexual characteristics and reproductive functions

CROSSWORD PUZZLE

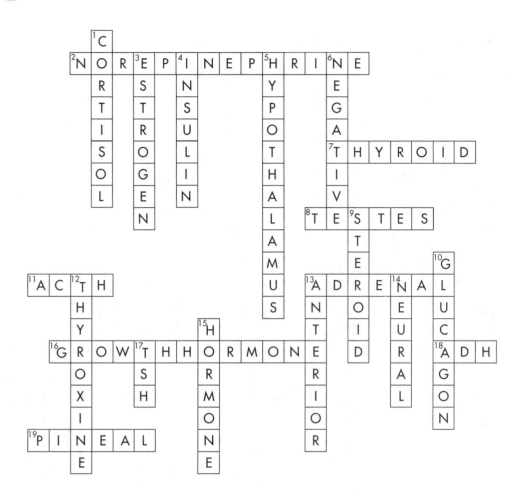

Across

2. sympathetic hormone
7. the _____ and parathyroid glands control calcium levels
8. secrete testosterone
11. stimulates adrenal cortex (abbreviation)
13. the _____ gland secretes steroid hormones
16. too little causes dwarfism (2 words)
18. abbreviation for hormone released from posterior pituitary
19. secretes melatonin

Down

1. stress hormone
3. released from ovaries
4. decreases blood sugar
5. controls pituitary gland
6. type of feedback involved in hormonal control
9. can cross cell membrane and interact directly with DNA
10. secreted when blood sugar drops
12. hormone that contains iodine
13. the _____ pituitary makes and secretes its own hormones
14. the release of epinephrine is under _____ control
15. chemical messenger released from endocrine glands
17. abbreviation for hormone that triggers release of T3 and T4

CONCEPT MAP

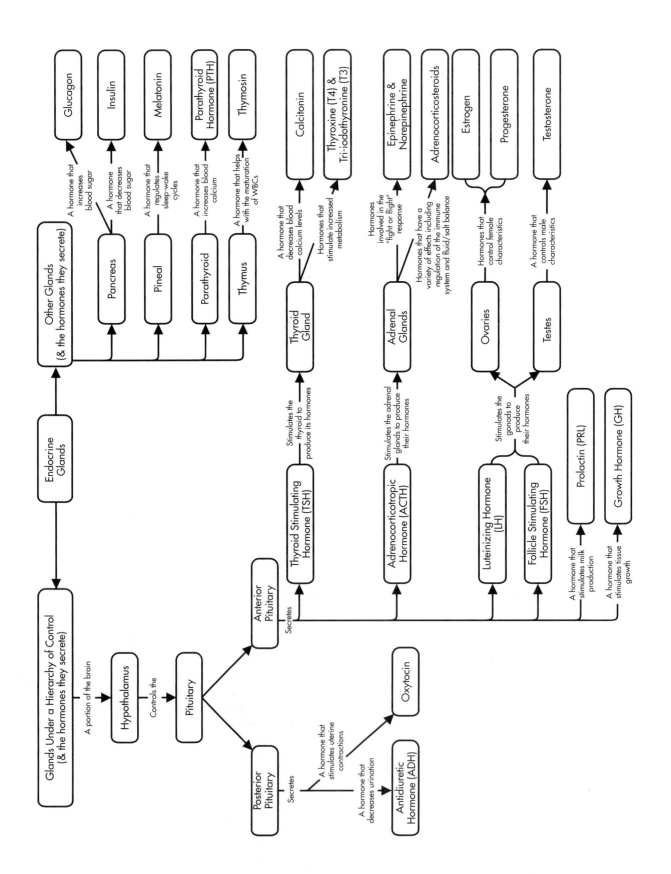

CHAPTER 13
ANSWER KEY

MEDICAL TERMINOLOGY REVIEW

1. Arteriosclerosis: Hardening of the arteries due to age, deposits, or degeneration
2. Thrombus: Blood clot
3. Embolus: Traveling blood clot
4. Leukemia: Cancer that causes overproduction of white blood cells
5. Myocardial infarct: Heart attack; decreased blood flow to heart tissue leads to ischemia; also called MI
6. Ischemia: Tissue injury caused by reduced blood flow
7. Aneurysm: Weakened area in blood vessel; may rupture causing serious hemorrhage
8. Anemia: Decreased oxygen-carrying capacity of blood due to decreased red blood cells or decreased hemoglobin
9. Atherosclerosis: Blockage of arteries by plaque
10. Arrhythmia: Irregular heartbeat

MULTIPLE CHOICE

1. b
2. b
3. d
4. d
5. b
6. b
7. c
8. c
9. a
10. b
11. b
12. c
13. a
14. c
15. a
16. a
17. b
18. d
19. c
20. d
21. a
22. c
23. b
24. b
25. d

MATCHING EXERCISES

Set 1	Set 2	Set 3	Set 4
1. i	1. d	1. f	1. f
2. f	2. c	2. j	2. a
3. h	3. f	3. a	3. h
4. d	4. i	4. g	4. j
5. g	5. j	5. h	5. c
6. a	6. h	6. i	6. d
7. b	7. e	7. b	7. b
8. c	8. a	8. e	8. g
9. j	9. g	9. d	9. e
10. e	10. b	10. c	10. i

FILL IN THE BLANK

1. away from
2. interventricular septum
3. QRS
4. gases/nutrients/wastes/hormones
5. formed elements/plasma
6. liver/K
7. interatrial septum
8. tricuspid or right AV
9. increase
10. right atrium
11. Calcium or Ca
12. fibrin
13. cholesterol
14. sphygmomanometer/stethoscope
15. inferior vena cava/superior vena cava
16. prehypertension
17. atherosclerosis
18. Arteriosclerosis
19. arrhythmia
20. anemia
21. polycythemia
22. capillaries
23. embolus
24. aneurysm
25. myocardial infarction

SHORT ANSWER

1. Agglutination is clumping of the surface antigens on the red blood cells. This is a potentially dangerous situation. Coagulation is clotting, usually at a site of injury, and it uses clotting proteins dissolved in the plasma as well as vitamin K. Clotting prevents blood loss when a vessel is compromised.

2. The vessel that leaves the right ventricle is called the pulmonary trunk, which leads to the pulmonary arteries. The arteries and the trunk itself route deoxygenated blood toward the lungs. Since it carries blood away from the heart, the vessels are termed *arteries*. The pulmonary veins, on the other hand, route blood from the lungs back to the heart. The blood is oxygen-rich. Since it approaches or leads to the heart, these vessels are termed *veins*. Fetal circulation follows the same principle.

3. Blood enters the right atrium via the superior and inferior vena cava. It flows through the tricuspid valve into the right ventricle then out the pulmonary semilunar valve through the pulmonary trunk (arteries) to the lungs. Blood comes back from the lungs via the pulmonary veins, to the left atrium, through the bicuspid valve to the left ventricle. Blood then flows from the left ventricle through the aortic semilunar valve out the aorta to the body.

4. Blood pressure is controlled by regulation of cardiac activity, peripheral resistance (size of blood vessels), and fluid volume. Increased cardiac activity, vasoconstriction, and increased fluid volume all increase BP. Anything that controls the heart, the size of blood vessels, or fluid volume can control blood pressure.

5. When a chamber contracts, pressure rises. When atria contract, pressure presses against the arioventricular valves (AV), opening the AV valves. When the ventricles contract, they push the AV valves closed and push the semilunar valves open.

LABELING ACTIVITY

This illustration should be color-coded per Figure 13–1 in the text.

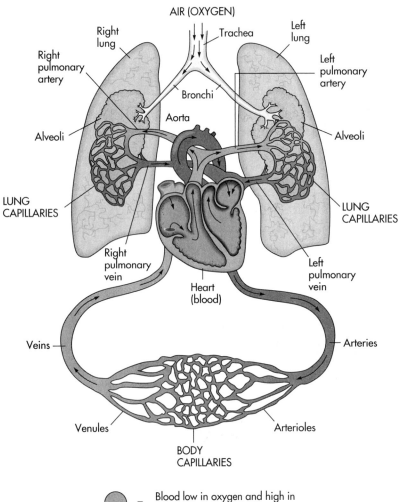

CROSSWORD PUZZLE

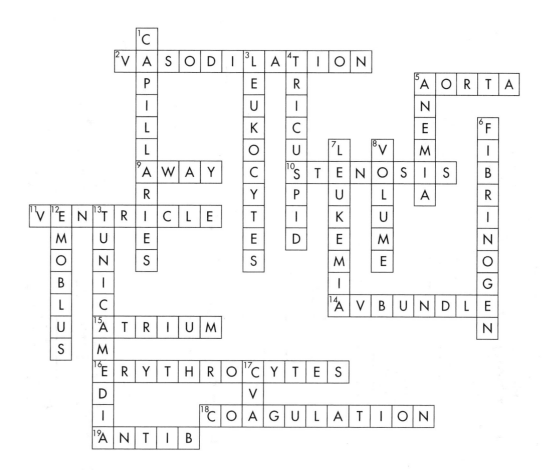

Across

2. decreases peripheral resistance
5. the vessel that carries blood from the left ventrical
9. arteries carry blood _____ from the heart
10. a narrowing of a valve is called _____
11. cardiac cycle refers to contraction of this chamber
14. impulse spreads from AV node to _____ (2 words)
15. superior vena cava empties into the right _____
16. red blood cells
18. clotting
19. type A blood has these antibodies (2 words)

Down

1. smallest blood vessels
3. technical term for white blood cells
4. the valve between the right atrium and ventricle
5. can be caused by decreased hemoglobin or RBCs
6. soluble fiber in platelet plug
7. cancer which results in large numbers of white blood cells
8. ADH controls BP by controlling blood _____
12. floating blood clot
13. layer of blood vessel innervated by sympathetic axons (2 words)
17. stroke abbreviation

CONCEPT MAP

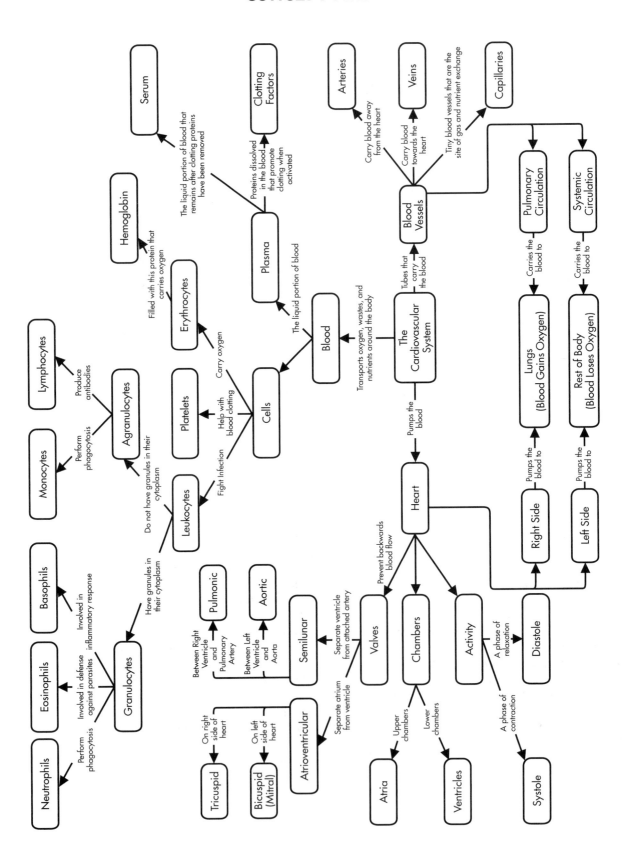

CHAPTER 14
ANSWER KEY

MEDICAL TERMINOLOGY REVIEW

1. Atelectasis: Collapsed lung
2. Emphysema: Nonreversible lung condition in which the alveolar air sacs are destroyed and the lung itself becomes "floppy"
3. Tuberculosis: Bacterial infection of lungs, may be dormant for several years; abbreviated TB
4. Pneumothorax: A condition in which there is air inside thoracic cavity and outside the lungs
5. Asthma: A potentially life-threatening lung condition in which the body reacts to an allergy by causing constriction of the airways of the lungs (bronchospasm), that leads to gas trapping because fresh air cannot get into the lungs, so the victim breathes the same air over and over
6. Ventilation: Bulk movement of air into and out of the lungs
7. Respiration: Gas exchange deep within the lungs, in which oxygen is added to the blood and carbon dioxide is removed
8. Chronic obstructive pulmonary disease: Group of diseases characterized by large amounts of secretions, lung damage, and difficult expiration; called COPD
9. Pleural effusion: Excessive buildup of fluid in pleural cavity between the parietal and the visceral pleura
10. Tidal volume: Amount of air moved during a single breath

MULTIPLE CHOICE

1. d
2. b
3. a
4. c
5. a
6. b
7. a
8. b
9. a
10. d
11. b
12. d
13. b
14. c
15. a
16. a
17. b
18. c
19. b
20. d
21. b
22. a
23. a
24. d
25. d

MATCHING EXERCISES

Set 1	Set 2	Set 3	Set 4
1. g	1. h	1. e	1. e
2. i	2. e	2. d	2. h
3. c	3. b	3. j	3. d
4. k	4. j	4. k	4. g
5. f	5. i	5. i	5. i
6. h	6. d	6. b	6. f
7. b	7. f	7. h	7. a
8. d	8. a	8. g	8. j
9. e	9. c	9. a	9. c
10. j	10. g	10. f	10. b

FILL IN THE BLANK

1. mucociliary
2. nasopharynx/oropharynx/larynopharynx
3. larynx
4. windpipe
5. conducting
6. hilum
7. diaphragm
8. 3, 2
9. alveoli
10. 12, 7, 2
11. apex
12. decreases
13. alveolar capillary membrane (respiratory membrane)
14. increase/increase
15. middle ear/pharynx
16. medulla oblongata
17. Carbon dioxide
18. aorta, carotids, medulla oblongata
19. smoking
20. right
21. phrenic
22. collapsed
23. emphysema
24. laryngitis
25. mucus

SHORT ANSWER

1. The diaphragm contracts, increasing thoracic and lung volume. That causes pressure to decrease, which allows air to flow into the lungs.

2. The primary functions of the respiratory system include bringing oxygen from the atmosphere into the bloodstream and removing carbon dioxide from the bloodstream.

3. Other muscles of inspiration include the external intercostals, sternocleidomastoid, scalenes, pectoralis major, and pectoralis minor that all pull the rib cage up, increasing the volume and decreasing the pressure. Inspiration then occurs.

4. Internal respiration is gas exchange between blood and body cells. Oxygen moves into the cells and carbon dioxide leaves the cells, moving into the blood capillaries. External respiration is the exchange of gases in the lungs where oxygen is moved from alveoli into the pulmonary capillaries, and carbon dioxide moves from the pulmonary capillaries into the alveoli.

5. Ventilation rate is determined by CO_2 blood levels. As CO_2 level rises, blood pH drops. That causes the ventilation rate to increase.

LABELING ACTIVITY

See Figure 14–1 in the textbook for comparison.

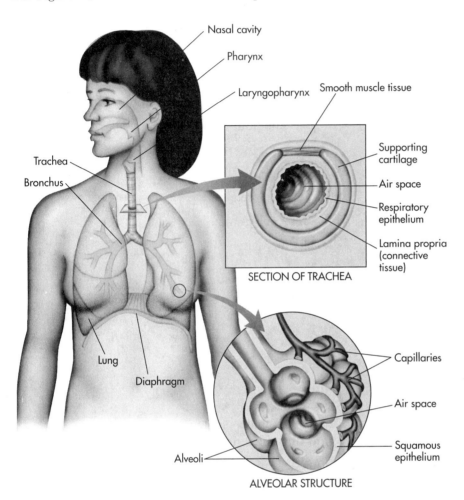

CROSSWORD PUZZLE

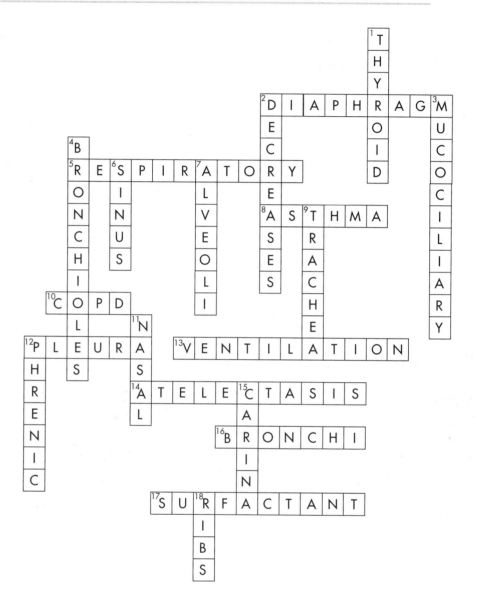

Across

2. the prime muscle of inspiration
5. zone of tracheobronchial tree where gas exchange occurs
8. breathing difficulty often triggered by allergies
10. group of disorders including emphysema and chronic bronchitis (abbreviation)
12. serous membrane in thoracic cavity
13. bulk movement of air into and out of respiratory system
14. collapse of alveoli
16. lobar _____, one in each lobe of each lung
17. may be missing or decreased in premature babies

Down

1. Adam's apple; _____ cartilage
2. when the diaphragm contracts, thoracic pressure _____
3. _____ escalator; cilia moving mucus
4. small airways
6. cavity in facial bone, connected to nasal cavity
7. air sacs
9. wind pipe
11. cavity posterior to nose
12. motor nerve for diaphragm
15. split of trachea into main bronchi
18. 12 pairs, part of thoracic cage

CONCEPT MAP

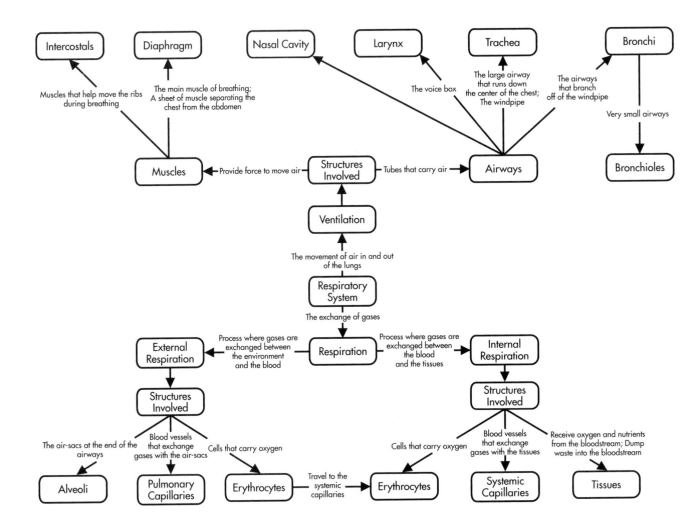

CHAPTER 15
ANSWER KEY

MEDICAL TERMINOLOGY REVIEW

1. Anaphylaxis: Widespread inflammation due to allergic reaction that causes vasodilation, low blood pressure, and can lead to shock
2. Cytokine: Proteins produced by damaged tissues and white blood cells that stimulate immune response by increasing inflammation, stimulating lymphocytes, and enhancing phagocytosis; involved in both innate and adaptive immunity
3. Antibody: A protein that binds to an antigen to inactivate it
4. Antigen: A cell surface protein used by the body for cell identification
5. Acquired immune deficiency syndrome: AIDS; immune system failure caused by infection of helper T cells by the human immunodeficiency virus
6. Autoimmune disorder: Disease in which the immune system attacks and destroys healthy body tissues
7. Innate immunity: Innate, inborn, nonspecific methods for defending against infection
8. Adaptive immunity: Acquired, specific response to pathogens that recognizes specific pathogens and improves with experience
9. Lymph node: Bean-shaped lymphatic filters
10. Leukemia: Cancer of white blood cells leading to abnormally high numbers of abnormal, usually malfunctioning, white blood cells

MULTIPLE CHOICE

1. a
2. d
3. a
4. a
5. d
6. d
7. c
8. a
9. a
10. d
11. c
12. b
13. b
14. b
15. d
16. b
17. b
18. d
19. c
20. a
21. d
22. b
23. d
24. b
25. d

MATCHING EXERCISES

Set 1
1. c
2. a
3. e
4. f
5. b
6. h
7. j
8. i
9. d
10. g

Set 2
1. b
2. a
3. c
4. d
5. h
6. i
7. g
8. j
9. f
10. e

Set 3
1. c
2. h
3. d
4. i
5. b
6. e
7. f
8. g
9. a
10. j

Set 4
1. h
2. e
3. a
4. d
5. j
6. b
7. c
8. f
9. i
10. g

Copyright © 2020 by Pearson Education, Inc.

FILL IN THE BLANK

1. allergy
2. lymphocytes/macrophages
3. positive selection
4. CD4 and CD8
5. proliferation
6. anaphylaxis/low
7. margination, increased WBC, increased fluid
8. Helper T
9. three
10. negative selection
11. lymphatic sinuses
12. histamine
13. inflammatory
14. helper T cells
15. cytokines
16. Helper T cells
17. lymphocytes
18. palatine, pharyngeal, lingual
19. Tumor necrosis factor
20. complement cascade
21. secondary
22. immune deficiency
23. mononuclear phagocyte (or reticuloendothelial)
24. skin, mucous membranes, hairs, tears, saliva
25. Immunosuppressant

SHORT ANSWER

1. Immune deficiency can be caused by genetics, chemicals, radiation exposure, or even medication. Immune-compromised clients include those with severe combined immune deficiency, a genetic disorder, leukemia, some forms of anemia, and patients undergoing chemotherapy or taking immune-suppressing drugs after organ transplant.

2. Lymph nodes filter lymph fluid and destroy pathogens with the WBCs that are housed in the nodes.

3. The spleen is structurally similar to lymph nodes, but instead of having lymphatic sinuses, the spleen has blood sinuses.

4. Innate immune mechanisms are triggered by the presence of foreign antigens in the body. They hold off the infection and stimulate adaptive immune mechanisms. Adaptive immunity uses T and B lymphocytes to fight specific pathogens. Lymphocytes must be selected during development to recognize foreign antigens and ignore the body's own antigens. Lymphocytes must be activated to fight a pathogen by binding with antigen-presenting cells, and then proliferate, making thousands of copies of themselves.

5. CD-4 cells are necessary for the proliferation of B cells and cytotoxic T cells.

LABELING ACTIVITY

See Figures 15-2 and 15-3 in the textbook for comparison.

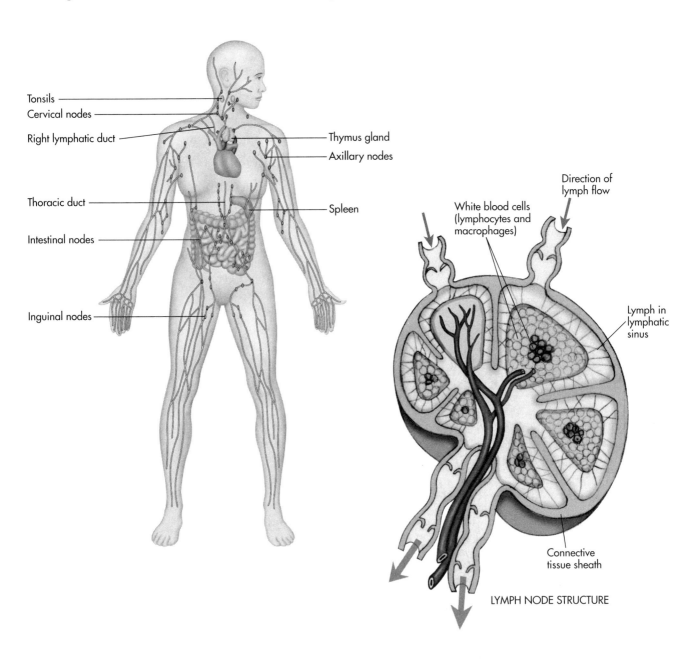

LYMPH NODE STRUCTURE

CROSSWORD PUZZLE

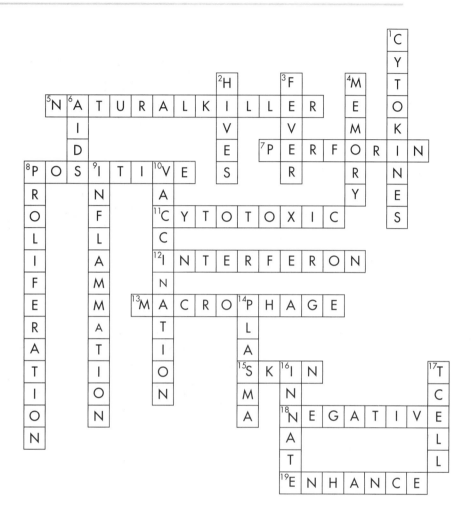

Across

5. _____ cells: the only lymphocytes in innate immunity (2 words)
7. chemical released by T cells for direct cell killing
8. selection for immune competent lymphocytes
11. _____ T cell; cell mediated immunity
12. protects cells from viral infection
13. antigen displaying cell
15. one of the body's physical barriers
18. selection against lymphocytes which react to self-antigens
19. antibodies and complement _____ phagocytosis

Down

1. chemicals which enhance immunity
2. skin response to hypersensitivity reaction
3. increased body temperature
4. _____ B cells mediate secondary response
6. full blown disorder caused by HIV
8. reproduction of activated lymphocytes
9. swelling, heat, redness, pain
10. deliberate exposure of patient to weakened or dead pathogen
14. B cell responsible for primary response
16. inborn, does not recognize specific pathogens
17. helper, cytotoxic, memory and regulatory for example (2 words)

CONCEPT MAP

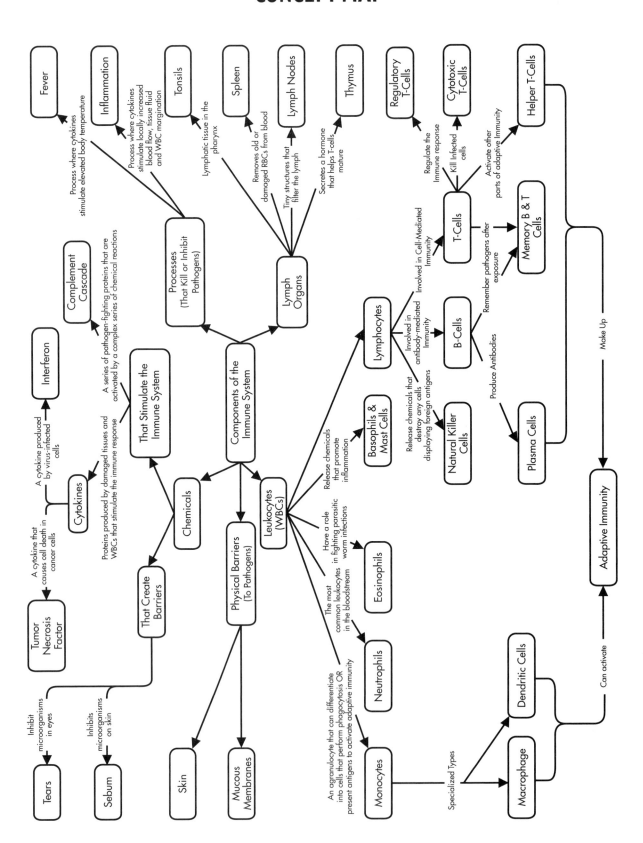

CHAPTER 16
ANSWER KEY

MEDICAL TERMINOLOGY REVIEW

1. Cholecystitis: Inflammation of the gallbladder
2. Pancreatitis: Inflammation of the pancreas
3. Hepatitis: Inflammation of the liver
4. Diverticulitis: Inflammation of a diverticulum or sac in the intestinal tract, especially in the colon
5. Gastroesophageal reflux disease: Backflow of stomach acid into esophagus; abbreviated GERD
6. Caries: Cavities in teeth caused by enamel destruction
7. Cirrhosis: Chronic liver disease that causes scarring of the liver
8. Gastroenteritis: Inflammation of the stomach and small intestine
9. Peptic ulcer: Wound (ulcer) in the lower portion of the esophagus, stomach, or duodenum thought to be caused by the acid of gastric juices, possibly initiated by bacterial infection
10. Ulcerative colitis: Ulceration of the mucous membranes of the colon of unknown origin; also known as inflammatory bowel disease (IBD)

MULTIPLE CHOICE

1. c
2. a
3. b
4. a
5. a
6. d
7. b
8. c
9. d
10. c
11. a
12. d
13. a
14. c
15. a
16. d
17. b
18. a
19. c
20. a
21. d
22. c
23. a
24. a
25. d

MATCHING EXERCISES

Set 1	Set 2	Set 3	Set 4
1. c	1. l/f	1. l	1. i
2. g	2. f/l	2. b	2. j
3. h	3. a	3. i	3. b
4. k	4. k	4. d	4. h
5. j	5. b	5. j	5. d
6. f	6. h	6. g	6. f
7. i	7. e	7. k	7. g
8. b	8. i	8. h	8. c
9. a	9. g	9. c	9. e
10. d	10. c	10. e	10. a

FILL IN THE BLANK

1. vestigial
2. cuspids
3. parasympathetic
4. visceral peritoneum
5. 20
6. defecation
7. alimentary
8. diarrhea
9. epiglottis
10. cecum/colon/rectum
11. pancreas/gallbladder
12. deciduous
13. cardiac sphincter
14. amylase
15. constipation
16. lactose
17. appendectomy
18. Hemorrhoids
19. liver
20. pancreas
21. hiatal hernia
22. Jaundice
23. stomach pain, diarrhea, nausea, constipation (students should list two of these)
24. retroperitoneal
25. smell (or taste, see, or think about)

SHORT ANSWER

1. Villi, plicae circulares, and microvilli provide an incredible increase in the surface area of the small intestine, which increases the effectiveness of the absorption of nutrients.

2. The cephalic phase occurs as a result of sensory stimulation, such as the sight, thought of, or smell of food. This sensory input stimulates the parasympathetic nervous system via the medulla oblongata, and the release of the hormone gastrin is increased. Gastric activity is increased. This leads to the gastric phase, in which over two-thirds of the gastric juices are secreted as the food moves into the stomach. As the food moves in, the stomach begins to distend. As the stomach distends, it sends signals back to the brain, which fires a reply to the gastric glands to step up their work. As chyme is formed, it is passed through the pyloric sphincter to the first part of the small intestine, the duodenum. This begins the intestinal phase of gastric juice regulation. As the duodenum distends and senses the acidity of chyme, intestinal hormones are released that cause the gastric glands in the stomach to decrease gastric juice production. The brain is also signaled and sends a message to inhibit gastric juice secretion because it is no longer needed now that the food bolus (now called chyme) has left the stomach.

3. The liver has many functions. It detoxifies (removes poisons) the body of harmful substances such as certain drugs and alcohol; destroys old blood cells; forms blood plasma proteins; produces the clotting factors fibrinogen and prothrombin; creates the anticoagulant heparin; manufactures bile; stores and modifies fats for more efficient usage by the body's cells; synthesizes urea, a by-product of protein metabolism, so it can be eliminated by the body; stores the simple sugar glucose as glycogen; stores iron and vitamins A, B12, D, E, and K; and produces cholesterol.

4. The digestive hormones and their functions include gastrin, which stimulates stomach activity; and cholecystokinin (CCK) and secretin, which decrease stomach activity, stimulate pancreas secretion, and stimulate bile release from the gall bladder and liver, respectively.

5. The accessory organs and their functions include the following: salivary glands secrete saliva, which moistens food and begins starch digestion. The liver secretes bile and has many other functions. The gallbladder stores bile. The pancreas secretes an alkaline fluid with enzymes.

LABELING ACTIVITY

See Figure 16–1 in the textbook for comparison.

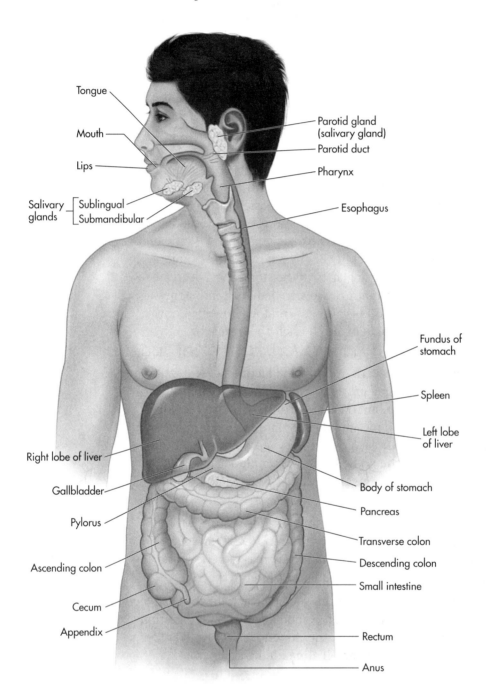

CROSSWORD PUZZLE

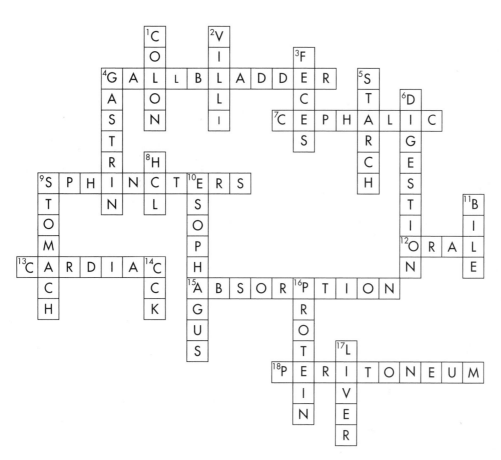

Across

4. stores bile
7. phase of gastric activity that begins before you even eat
9. valves between parts of alimentary canal
12. starch is digested in this cavity
13. part of stomach connected to esophagus
15. small intestine does almost all of this
18. serous membrane lining abdominal cavity

Down

1. medical term for large intestine
2. projections that increase surface area of small intestine
3. stored in large intestine
4. increases stomach activity
5. digested by amylase
6. breakdown of food into nutrients
8. acid in stomach (abbreviation)
9. stores food
10. no digestion takes place here
11. emulsifier
14. decreases stomach activity (abbreviation)
16. digestion begins in stomach
17. detoxification organ

CONCEPT MAP

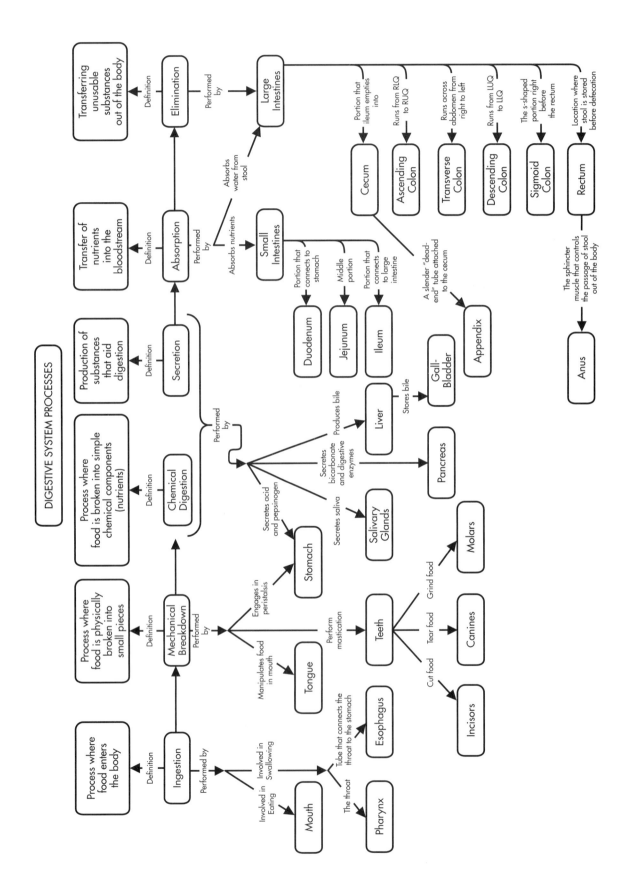

CHAPTER 17
ANSWER KEY

MEDICAL TERMINOLOGY REVIEW

1. Polycystic kidney disease: Genetic disorder in which large cysts develop in the kidneys; abbreviated PKD
2. Diabetic nephropathy: Kidney damage caused by diabetes mellitus
3. Glomerulonephritis: Inflammation of the glomerulus
4. Glomerulosclerosis: Scarring of the glomerulus
5. Analgesic nephropathy: Kidney damage caused by overuse or abuse of drugs
6. Lithotripsy: Using shockwaves to break up a kidney stone
7. Renal failure: Kidney disease, decreased kidney function
8. Ischemia: A condition of tissue injury resulting from too little oxygen delivery to tissues, usually caused by decreased blood flow
9. Creatinine: Waste product of muscle metabolism
10. Antidiuretic hormone: Hormone made by the hypothalamus and secreted from the posterior pituitary when blood pressure decreases or blood ionic concentration increases; abbreviated ADH.

MULTIPLE CHOICE

1. a
2. d
3. b
4. a
5. b
6. c
7. b
8. a
9. c
10. b
11. b
12. c
13. b
14. c
15. d
16. a
17. b
18. a
19. c
20. c
21. d
22. b
23. c
24. a
25. a

MATCHING EXERCISES

Set 1	Set 2	Set 3	Set 4
1. b	1. e	1. d	1. f
2. f	2. c	2. e	2. j
3. i	3. h	3. a	3. a
4. g	4. d	4. j	4. d
5. a	5. i	5. b	5. i
6. e	6. j	6. g	6. b
7. h	7. f	7. c	7. g
8. j	8. g	8. i	8. c
9. c	9. b	9. h	9. h
10. d	10. a	10. f	10. e

FILL IN THE BLANK

1. filtration/secretion/reabsorption
2. afferent arterioles/efferent arterioles
3. renal corpuscle/renal tubule
4. alcohol
5. lithotripsy
6. diabetic nephropathy
7. aldosterone
8. diabetes mellitus
9. renal vein/ureter/renal artery
10. renal pelvis
11. nephron
12. descending limb (nephron loop)
13. secretion
14. Renin
15. parasympathetic
16. renal capsule
17. creatinine
18. blood
19. pons
20. Polycystic kidney disease
21. HCO_3^- (bicarbonate ions)
22. hemolytic uremic syndrome
23. excessive urination
24. hydrogen ions
25. ischemia

SHORT ANSWER

1. Urinary tract infections are more common in women than men because a woman's urethra is shorter than a man's and fecal matter can more easily travel to the urinary bladder and up the urinary tract.

2. As systemic blood pressure increases over normal range of BP, and the afferent arterioles leading into the glomerulus constrict, decreasing the amount of blood getting into the glomerulus. Autoregulation protects the delicate filters from repeated rapid changes in blood pressure.

3. If there is too much acid in the blood, hydrogen ions, which cause acidity and the pH to drop, will be excreted to a greater level in the urine. At the same time, more bicarbonate ions will be reabsorbed back into the acidic blood, pulling the pH up to a more neutral level.

4. Aldosterone increases the reabsorption of sodium. In contrast, atrial natriuretic hormone decreases sodium reabsorption.

5. With massive blood loss, blood pressure falls. To maintain normal blood pressure, there is widespread vasoconstriction. The afferent arterioles of the kidneys get smaller, greatly decreasing blood supply to the nephrons. Tissues soon become ischemic and begin to die.

LABELING ACTIVITY

See Figure 16–2 in the textbook for comparison.

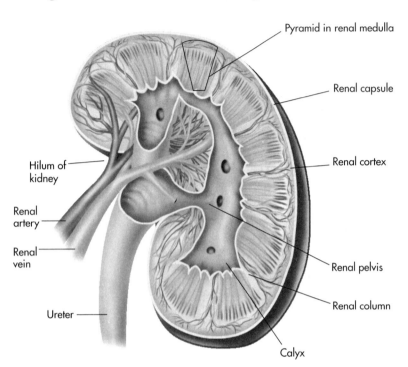

CROSSWORD PUZZLE

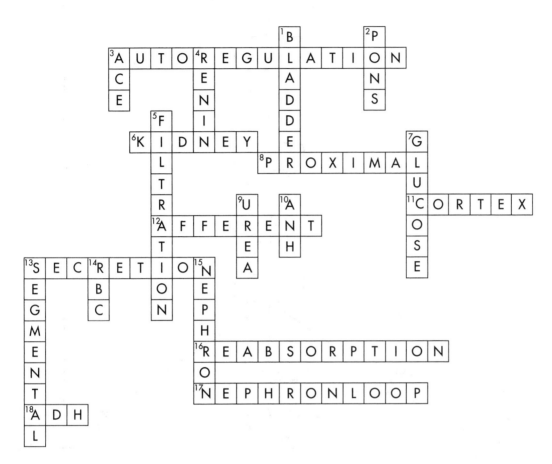

Across

3. protects glomerulus from typical blood pressure changes
6. organs that control fluid and ion balance
8. tubule where most reabsorption and secretion takes place
11. outer layer of kidney, where filters are
12. arteriole leading to glomerulus
13. movement of substances from capillaries into tubule
16. movement of substances into bloodstream from tubules
17. where countercurrent circulation takes place (2 words)
18. made in hypothalamus, decreases urine production; abbreviation

Down

1. urinary _____ stores urine
2. part of brain which controls urination
3. enzyme which regulates blood pressure, abbreviation
4. secreted by kidney when blood flow decreases
5. movement of substances into kidney from blood at glomerulus
7. presence in urine is indicator of diabetes
9. nitrogen containing waste molecule
10. hormone which increases urine output; abbreviation
13. missing kidney vein
14. cannot normally pass through filter, abbreviation
15. fundamental functional unit of kidney

CONCEPT MAP

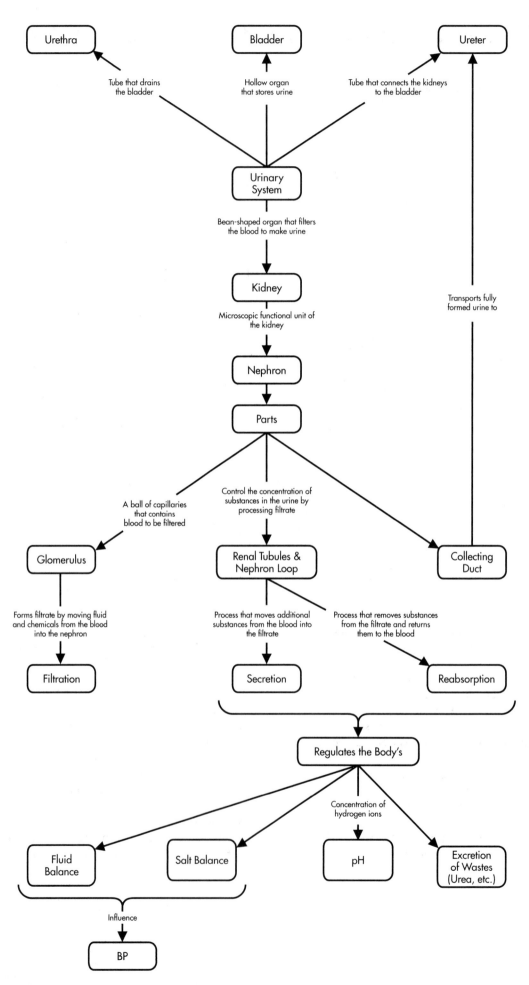

CHAPTER 18
ANSWER KEY

MEDICAL TERMINOLOGY REVIEW

1. Endometriosis: Implantation of endometrial tissue outside the uterus where it sheds each month with the woman's menstrual cycle, causing pain and scarring
2. Amenorrhea: Absence of a menstrual cycle
3. Ectopic pregnancy: Implantation of embryo in the wrong place, usually in the fallopian tubes; also called tubal pregnancy
4. Cryptorchidism: Testes fail to descend into the scrotal sac during development
5. Erectile dysfunction disorder: The inability to initiate or maintain erection; abbreviated EDD
6. Benign prostatic hyperplasia: Enlargement of the prostate that is not cancerous; abbreviated BPH
7. Hydrocele: Abnormal collection of fluid in testes
8. Androgen insensitivity: Genetic disorder in which tissues do not respond to testosterone
9. Prostate cancer: Uncontrolled spread of prostate cells, causing prostate enlargement
10. Premenstrual syndrome: Physical and psychological symptoms related to a woman's menstrual cycle; abbreviated PMS

MULTIPLE CHOICE

1. c
2. c
3. d
4. a
5. b
6. b
7. c
8. a
9. a
10. c
11. d
12. c
13. b
14. a
15. d
16. b
17. a
18. d
19. c
20. c
21. a
22. a
23. d
24. b
25. a

MATCHING EXERCISES

Set 1	Set 2	Set 3	Set 4
1. d	1. c	1. d	1. d
2. j	2. g	2. j	2. h
3. e	3. h	3. e	3. a
4. f	4. a	4. f	4. i
5. b	5. i	5. b	5. b
6. a	6. j	6. a	6. g
7. g	7. f	7. g	7. j
8. h	8. b	8. h	8. c
9. i	9. e	9. i	9. f
10. c	10. d	10. c	10. e

FILL IN THE BLANK

1. XX/XY
2. semen/urine
3. spermatogenesis
4. erection
5. alveoli
6. pudendal
7. luteal
8. seminal vesicles
9. eukaryotic
10. pituitary gland
11. foreskin
12. fundus
13. testes
14. before birth (in utero)
15. cervix
16. pap test
17. fallopian tubes
18. 46, zygote
19. benign prostatic hypertrophy and prostate cancer
20. placenta
21. vasectomy
22. negative
23. luteinizing hormone
24. human chorionic gonadotropin
25. Progesterone

SHORT ANSWER

1. The first menstrual period is called the menarche, and menopause represents the ending of menstrual activity.

2. The three stages of labor are the dilation, delivery, and placenta stages. The dilation stage is when contraction of the uterine smooth muscle is noted and the cervix also dilates to allow passage of the fetus's head. The delivery stage is noted with the presenting of the fetus's head, called *crowning*. The mouth is suctioned at this stage. The placenta stage is when the placenta or afterbirth is delivered with the final uterine contraction.

3. Estrogen stimulates the proliferation of the uterine lining, and progesterone maintains the buildup of the endometrium.

4. The 23rd pair of chromosomes is the sex chromosomes. These are called sex chromosomes because their identity determines the sex of a baby. XX is female and XY is male. The female always contributes an X, but the male can contribute either an X or Y chromosome. The male actually determines the sex of the baby by contributing either an X chromosome for a girl or a Y chromosome for a boy.

5. Sperm are propelled from the epididymis of the scrotal sac into the vas deferens, which then carries the sperm into the pelvic cavity. As the sperm pass the seminal vesicles, sugar and chemicals are added to the sperm, then the substance enters the ejaculatory duct. As the ejaculatory duct passes through the prostate gland, prostatic fluid is added, liquefying the semen. The semen passes by the bulbourethral glands, which add mucus to the semen. The semen is then released into the vagina.

LABELING ACTIVITY

See Figure 5–17 in the textbook for comparison.

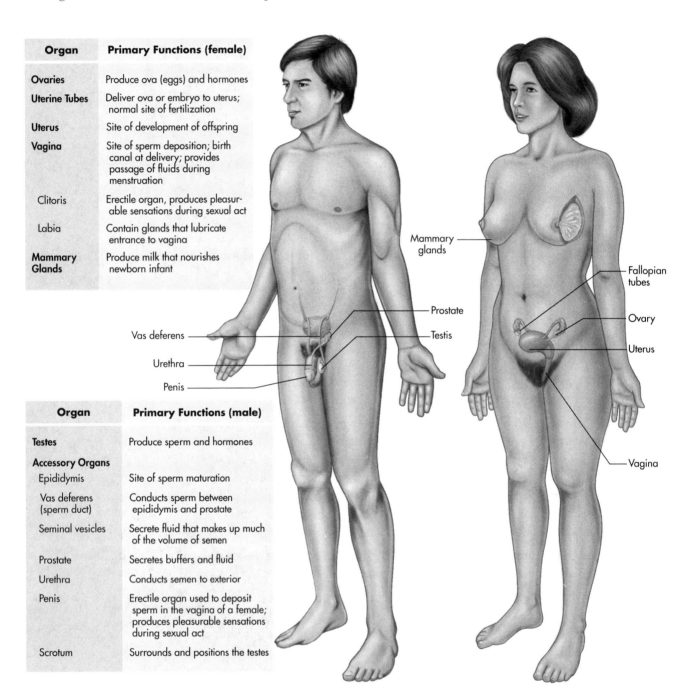

Organ	Primary Functions (female)
Ovaries	Produce ova (eggs) and hormones
Uterine Tubes	Deliver ova or embryo to uterus; normal site of fertilization
Uterus	Site of development of offspring
Vagina	Site of sperm deposition; birth canal at delivery; provides passage of fluids during menstruation
Clitoris	Erectile organ, produces pleasurable sensations during sexual act
Labia	Contain glands that lubricate entrance to vagina
Mammary Glands	Produce milk that nourishes newborn infant

Organ	Primary Functions (male)
Testes	Produce sperm and hormones
Accessory Organs	
Epididymis	Site of sperm maturation
Vas deferens (sperm duct)	Conducts sperm between epididymis and prostate
Seminal vesicles	Secrete fluid that makes up much of the volume of semen
Prostate	Secretes buffers and fluid
Urethra	Conducts semen to exterior
Penis	Erectile organ used to deposit sperm in the vagina of a female; produces pleasurable sensations during sexual act
Scrotum	Surrounds and positions the testes

CROSSWORD PUZZLE

Across

3. union of sperm and egg
6. stiffening of penis
7. _____ test, test for cervical cancer
8. female external genitalia
12. movement of fluid and tissue down the vagina
15. stimulates maturation of gametes
18. stimulate uterine contractions
19. controls development of female secondary sexual characters

Down

1. sperm delivery organ
2. birth canal
4. female primary genitalia
5. time during which a woman is menstruating
6. ejection of sperm from penis
9. where fertilized egg implants
10. layer of endometrium that is shed each month
11. secretes progesterone after ovulation
13. male primary genitalia
14. can be enlarged in older men
16. fertilized egg
17. stimulates secretion of FSH and LH

Copyright © 2020 by Pearson Education, Inc.

CONCEPT MAP

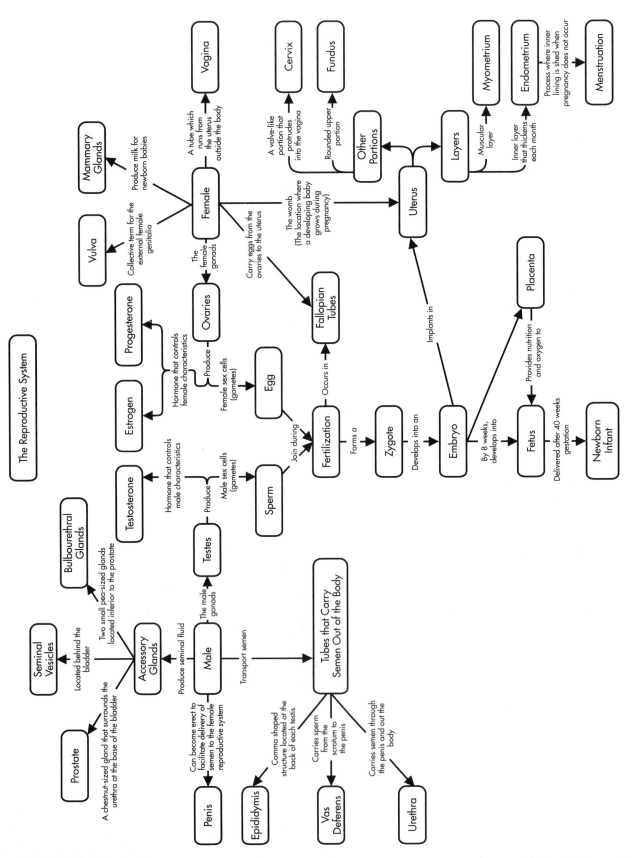

CHAPTER 19
ANSWER KEY

MEDICAL TERMINOLOGY REVIEW

1. DNA fingerprinting: Splitting DNA into fragments to compare an unknown sample to a known sample for identification
2. Geriatric: Pertaining to older patients
3. Polypharmacy: Taking many drugs at the same time
4. Chemotherapy: The use of chemicals to destroy rapidly dividing cells; used to treat cancer
5. Radiation: The use of energy waves to target cancer cells
6. Immunotherapy: Manipulating the body's immune system to defend itself against cancer
7. Sexually transmitted infection: Condition caused by pathogens that are spread by sexual contact; abbreviated STI
8. Melanoma: A potentially deadly form of skin cancer in which pigmented cells divide out of control
9. Colonoscopy: Screening technique for colon cancer using an endoscope to view the colon
10. Drug compliance: Taking drugs as directed

MULTIPLE CHOICE

1. a
2. a
3. a
4. d
5. a
6. b
7. c
8. c
9. b
10. b
11. d
12. d
13. d
14. c
15. d
16. d
17. c
18. a
19. d
20. c
21. b
22. b
23. d
24. b
25. c

MATCHING EXERCISES

Set 1	Set 2	Set 3	Set 4
1. c	1. g	1. j	1. f
2. d	2. a	2. d	2. i
3. g	3. h	3. f	3. b
4. h	4. b	4. g	4. h
5. j	5. i	5. b	5. a
6. b	6. c	6. e	6. c
7. e	7. j	7. i	7. d
8. i	8. d	8. h	8. j
9. a	9. e	9. c	9. g
10. f	10. f	10. a	10. e

FILL IN THE BLANK

1. Egyptians
2. thicker, drier
3. polypharmacy
4. 50
5. 35
6. muscle mass/bone density/fat
7. cervix
8. testosterone
9. breast
10. 450,000
11. radiation
12. sentinel lymph node mapping and biopsy
13. emphysema/bronchitis/asthma
14. congenital insensitivity to pain and anhidrosis
15. hair
16. elite
17. pain
18. renal
19. geriatric
20. A
21. resistance
22. natural sources
23. heart disease or diabetes mellitus
24. homeostasis
25. cancer

SHORT ANSWER

1. Cauliflowerlike growths on the penis and vagina.

2. Minimize time in the sun between 10 a.m. and 4 p.m.; wear long-sleeved shirt, brimmed hat, sunglasses, SPF sunscreen.

3. Kidney damage, liver damage, increased risk of heart disease, irritability, and aggressive behavior—all attributed to steroid abuse.

4. Changes in personality, such as becoming agitated, quiet, withdrawn, sad, confused, depressed, or grumpy, and behavior such as crying, swearing, grunting, loss of appetite, and wincing.

5. The acidic tomatoes served on pewter plates leached out the lead, which was consumed and led to lead poisoning.

CROSSWORD PUZZLE

```
              ¹S  T  ²D
              M     N
              O     A
          ³H  ⁴L  K
⁵F ⁶I N G ⁷E R P R I N T I N ⁸G
   N     A     V     F     N  E
   C     R           E     G  R
   O     L           S        I
   N     Y           T        A
   T     D  ⁹F       Y  ¹⁰S T R E S S
¹¹H A I R  E  O      L     R
   N     T  R     ¹²F      I
   E     E  E        R     C
   N  ¹³C A N C E R  I
   C     T     S     C
   E     I     I     T  ¹⁴P ¹⁵B  ¹⁶D
         O     C     ¹⁷S P I N A B I F I D A
         N           E  O  I  T  E
                     X  N  N  T  T
                              E
                  ¹⁸P O L Y P H A R M A C Y
```

Across

1. abbreviation, sexually transmitted disease
5. comparing one DNA sample to another is DNA _____
10. a little is healthy, but chronic is bad
11. can be a timeline of chemical exposure
13. the uncontrolled reproductionn and spread of abnormal cells
17. birth defect that can be prevented by vitamin B supplements (2 words)
18. taking many drugs at the same time

Down

1. millions of lives could be saved if people quit _____
2. the genetic material is in this molecule
3. virus that causes many cases of cervical cancer (abbreviation)
4. _____ choices have profound health effects
6. many older people suffer this uninary system disorder
7. many cancer deaths can be prevented by _____ (2 words)
8. referring to the elderly
9. _____ science is the application of science to crime
12. fingerprints are _____ ridges
14. many older patients are undermedicated for _____
15. this taste increases in intensity with age
16. becoming healthy involves changes in _____ and exercise
17. the _____ of the victim is often obvious from the pelvis

Copyright © 2020 by Pearson Education, Inc.

CONCEPT MAP

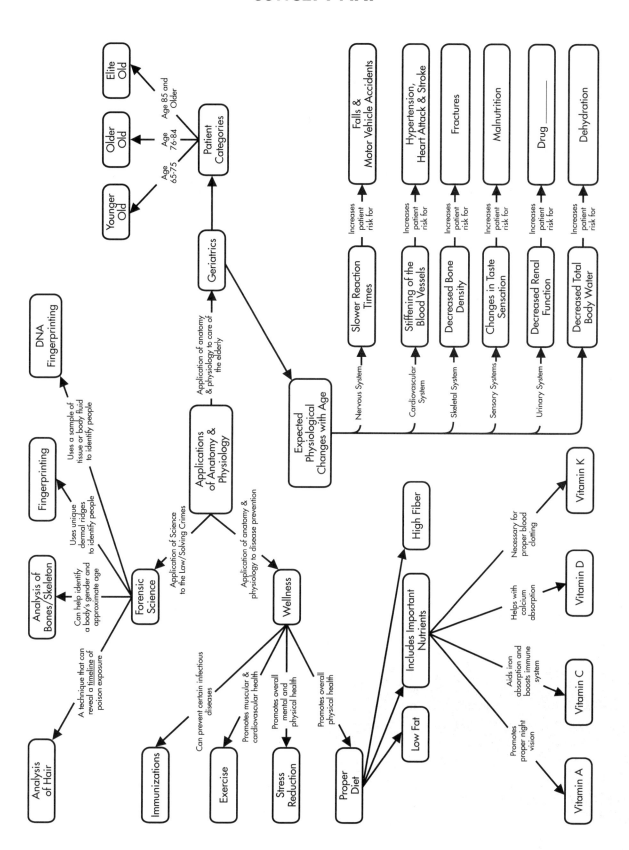